Anti Inflammatory Diet

FOR BEGINNERS

2 Books in 1

THE SECRET TO HEALTH!

Boost Your Immune System, Reactivate Your
Metabolism, Lose Weight Healthily, and Reduce
Inflammation

Jenni Serges

Thank you!

Life, at times, turns out to be a force that shapes our destiny in ways we can hardly imagine. At 27, my existence was shattered by a cancer diagnosis. This event marked not only a battle for survival but also the beginning of a journey of transformation and discovery. It was thanks to my oncologist that I approached the anti-inflammatory diet, a regime that I found supportive during the tough sessions of chemotherapy. After extensive research and collaboration closely with doctors, this dietary regime continues to be an integral part of my life after many years. Along my path, I have involved and provided advice to people who, wishing to gain health benefits, wanted to change their diet, just as I did. The anti-inflammatory diet proved to be not only an ally in managing cancer but also a source of vitality and well-being. The greatest challenge I faced was accepting the reality of cancer, a blow as devastating as a punch in the face. Despite this, I learned that resilience and the ability to rise from difficulties are what truly matter. Facing cancer is a constant struggle, a journey of highs and lows where the important thing is to never give up, always moving forward one step at a time. Reflecting on life, I often tell myself that nothing happens by chance and that even in the most adverse circumstances, we can find sprouts of hope. I thank every day for still being here, alive; and when I look up at the sky, my thoughts go to all the wonderful people I have met along this path and who, unfortunately, life has torn away from me. I am honored to have shared the fight with them and to have received a piece of their courage and heart. I am immensely grateful to my family: to the first man I loved, my father, who now watches over me like an angel from heaven, Thank you; to the second man in my life, my husband, whom I love more than my own existence, Thank you; to the women in my life, my mother and my sisters, I love you so much, Thank you. And to all other people, relatives, friends, doctors, and particularly to my super oncologist who has supported and tolerated me, I hold you dear, Thank you. Life can be long or painfully short, but the essential thing is to live it with all of ourselves, fully embracing who we are. It is this awareness that inspired me to write this book, hoping to offer not only advice and culinary inspiration but also an experience of exploration and satisfaction. Let's hold tight to what we have, Long live Life.

TABLE OF CONTENTS

YOUR FREE GIFT!!!

As a health enthusiast, you know the importance of attention to detail when it comes to improving your well-being. That's why I'm excited to present an exclusive bonus that complements your anti-inflammatory lifestyle journey. This bonus is an air fryer cookbook that exclusively uses anti-inflammatory foods, specifically designed to help you enjoy healthy and delicious meals with ease. This book covers everything from essential ingredients to creative recipe modifications, all designed to minimize inflammation and maximize health benefits. Modern cooking methods like air frying allow you not to sacrifice taste for health. With these new techniques, you can enjoy the full flavors of your meals while adhering to an anti-inflammatory diet.

Simply scan the provided QR code, and you will be well on your way to mastering the preparation and benefits of using your air fryer with anti-inflammatory foods. I'm here to make your journey towards health enriching and enjoyable.

Scan me

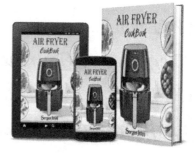

Preface

First and foremost, I want to thank you for choosing this book and deciding to embark on this culinary journey full of flavors, colors, and health benefits. I cannot express enough gratitude for your trust. These pages are divided into two parts, each dedicated to a fundamental aspect of the anti-inflammatory diet. In the first part, we will explore the essence of the anti-inflammatory diet: we will understand the foods to praise and those to avoid, learn how this diet can help us reduce inflammation and regenerate the body, and discover how it can be a valuable tool for preventing various diseases. Furthermore, we will explore the concept of Mindful Eating, a conscious approach to eating that will help us connect with food in a healthy and balanced way. Finally, you will find a 21-day meal plan designed to guide you through this transformative experience. The second part of the book is dedicated to recipes and their benefits. You will discover a wide selection of healthy, tasty, and nutritious recipes, designed to satisfy your tastes, and preserve the pleasure of the palate. Each recipe has been chosen for its contribution to your health and well-being. You will find dishes that enhance anti-inflammatory ingredients, but without sacrificing flavor and variety. The goal of this book is to demonstrate that eating healthily does not mean giving up taste, variety, or the satisfaction of a good meal. Through the recipes contained in these pages, I wish to share with you my belief that the kitchen can be a place of joy, creativity, and self-care. I hope that, as you go through these pages, you will find not only culinary inspiration but also a sense of discovery and fulfillment. May each of these recipes become a way for you to nourish both body and soul, exploring new flavors and enriching your life with delicious moments of pleasure. With gratitude and affection, I wish you enjoyable reading and a wonderful journey into the world of healthy cooking.

***Quote:** "Take care of your body. It's the only place you have to live." - Jim Rohn*

CHAPTER 1

"Lifetime Awakening: Reignite Your Health with the Anti-Inflammatory Diet"

The journey towards a healthier and more energetic life is within reach, thanks to the wonderful world of the anti-inflammatory diet. This diet is not just a simple eating plan, but a philosophy of life that transforms food into a powerful ally for our health.

The anti-inflammatory diet has the ambitious goal of reducing inflammation at the cellular level, a process that can cause diseases if left unchecked. It's like a firefighter extinguishing fires before they become disasters, pacifying the inflammatory processes that can threaten our health in the long term.

This diet goes beyond mere disease prevention. It is a journey of discovery and connection with a wide variety of nutritious and delicious foods. It is an invitation to embrace an abundance of flavors, colors, and textures, turning every meal into an opportunity to nourish the body and soul.

But it's not just about what we put on our plate. The anti-inflammatory diet also encompasses a healthy lifestyle and regular physical activity. It's a holistic approach to wellbeing, integrating nutrition, movement, and stress management to achieve a complete balance between body and mind.

Are you ready to embark on this exciting adventure? It doesn't matter where you come from or how old you are: the journey towards the anti-inflammatory diet is open to everyone. It's your ticket to a healthier and more fulfilling life, with the power to transform food into medicine and meals into acts of love towards yourself. Embark on this journey and discover how the anti-inflammatory diet can light up the path to your health.

Now, let's address the profound connection between the food we consume and our overall well-being. The plate we set before ourselves at every meal can be a minefield or a lush garden. It's all about making wise choices, because, in truth, every bite counts.

Picture it as a theater, where leading actors and extras play roles in the performance of our well-being. Some 'actors', like refined sugars, processed vegetable oils, highly processed foods, and red meats, can be the protagonists of a plot that does no good to our body. They have the ability to trigger the immune system's alarm, leading to a reaction that can cause tissue damage.

On the other hand, imagine food acting as a peacemaker, a mediator that promotes harmony in your body. These 'mediators', which include colorful fruits and vegetables, whole grains, fatty fish, nuts, and seeds, are the pillars of a healthy diet. These foods operate discreetly, silently supporting your well-being while you enjoy their delicious taste.

But how can a mere bite trigger or quell a storm in your body? Well, what you eat directly interacts with your gut, an organ that is increasingly emerging as the control center of well-being. A diet filled with 'problem actors' can disrupt the balance of bacteria in your gut, potentially triggering a chain reaction that involves the entire body. On the other hand, nourishing your body with 'mediators' can promote a healthy gut microbiota, which can keep your body running like a well-oiled machine.

So, here lies the wonder of a wellness-oriented diet. It might seem a bit like magic, but it's pure science. Consuming foods full of nutrients and antioxidants could be the key to maintaining optimal health, allowing you to live your life to the fullest.

It's important to remember that no food is inherently 'bad'. As with all things, moderation is key. But armed with knowledge and a dash of curiosity, you have the power to build a plate that not only satisfies but also nourishes.

Think of your next meal as an opportunity. An opportunity to nourish, to heal, to renew. It's a chance to celebrate the marvel of food and its powerful connection to our health. Because, in the end, we truly are what we eat.

Imagine being able to climb a mountain without stopping, to play with your kids without getting tired, to wake up in the morning feeling revitalized and ready to face the day. This is the promise of the eating habit we're talking about, a way of living that can reignite your energy potential like never before.

One of the first benefits you might notice is indeed an increase in energy. This isn't just a side effect of eating better, but also the result of reduced inflammation inside your body. When your body isn't constantly engaged in fighting inflammation, you have more energy resources available for daily activities. It's like having an engine running at full power, ready to take on every challenge.

You might also notice a reduction in pain, especially if you suffer from inflammation-related conditions such as arthritis. Some foods can act as natural pain relievers, helping to alleviate discomfort. It's a bit like having a personal masseuse available 24/7, working to reduce tension and pain.

But perhaps one of the most significant benefits is the boosting of your immune system. Your body has an extraordinary ability to heal and protect itself, but it needs the right fuel to do so. With a diet full of foods rich in antioxidants and nutrients, you are providing your body with the tools it needs to fend off diseases and keep you healthy. It's like equipping yourself with an invisible shield, ready to protect you from any threat.

This eating style doesn't just promise short-term benefits. Think of it as a long-term investment in your health. Every bite, every meal, is a step towards a healthier and happier future. It's a life insurance that doesn't require expensive premiums, only the willingness to make healthier choices every day.

You're not just adopting a new way of eating; you're embarking on a journey. There will be ups and downs, but every step brings you closer to optimal health. And the beauty of this journey is that it's unique to each of us.

Imagine holding a detailed map of gastrointestinal health in your hands. Each path on this map represents a key aspect of our digestive system, and your choice of foods can have a significant impact on each pathway.

Let's start with digestion. This complex process begins the moment we put food in our mouth. Some foods, like those high in fiber found in fruits, vegetables, and whole grains, can facilitate passage through the digestive system, contributing to a more comfortable digestion process.

There are multiple challenges along the way. Gastrointestinal disorders, such as irritable bowel syndrome or Inflammatory Bowel Disease, can create significant obstacles. Here, your diet can be a powerful ally. Foods that help reduce inflammation, like colorful fruits and vegetables, omega-3 fats found in fatty fish and seeds, can help soothe inflammation, easing symptoms and improving quality of life.

But the map doesn't stop here. A crucial aspect of gastrointestinal health involves nutrient absorption. It's not enough to simply consume nutrients; they must be properly absorbed to provide your body with the benefits they promise. Foods rich in probiotics, like yogurt and sauerkraut, and foods with fermentable fiber, like garlic and onions, can promote a healthy gut flora, enhancing nutrient assimilation.

This journey through gastrointestinal health shows how your diet can directly influence your well-being. Your food choices can become a powerful strategy for health, helping you navigate through challenges and making the most of the benefits along the way.

Your gastrointestinal health is a key indicator of your overall well-being. Nourishing your gut is like nourishing your body, laying the foundation for a healthier life. And with the right food choices, you can chart the most effective path on your personal health map.

Now let's talk about gastric reflux, a common condition characterized by the backflow of stomach acids into the esophagus, causing a burning sensation known as heartburn. The consumption of certain foods can often worsen symptoms, while others can help control them.

Starting a journey with the anti-inflammatory diet can make a difference in managing reflux. Fatty, spicy, or acidic foods, as well as caffeinated or alcoholic beverages, can increase stomach acidity, aggravating symptoms. On the contrary, foods like whole grains, leafy green vegetables, ginger root, and chamomile-based drinks can help soothe irritation.

The frequency and portions of meals can also affect reflux. Eating small amounts more frequently throughout the day, avoiding lying down immediately after a meal, can reduce pressure on the stomach and minimize the backflow of acids.

Thus, it not only helps promote overall intestinal health but can also provide tools to manage specific gastrointestinal disorders like gastric reflux. Listen to your body and adapt the diet to your personal needs.

The anti-inflammatory diet offers a number of significant benefits in the context of cancer prevention and nutrition during therapies, but it's important to emphasize that it represents a complement and does not replace traditional medicine in the treatment of diseases.

Numerous studies have highlighted the importance of a balanced diet rich in anti-inflammatory foods in reducing the risk of developing various forms of cancer. Anti-inflammatory foods, such as fruits, vegetables, whole grains, legumes, and spices, are rich in nutrients and antioxidants that can help combat chronic inflammation in the body, one of the risk factors for the development of several diseases, including cancer.

Furthermore, an anti-inflammatory diet can provide nutritional support during cancer therapies. Treatments such as chemotherapy and radiation therapy can cause side effects that affect appetite, digestion, and nutrient absorption. An anti-inflammatory diet, based on nutritious and easily digestible foods, can help maintain proper nutrition throughout the treatment journey.

It can contribute to reducing overall inflammation in the body, providing an unfavorable environment for the growth of cancer cells. Moreover, proper nutrition can help reduce the risk of recurrence and promote a better quality of life during and after treatment.

It's crucial to emphasize that the anti-inflammatory diet is just one element of a comprehensive approach to disease prevention and treatment. Following the advice of qualified health professionals, such as doctors and dietitians, to develop a personalized dietary plan based on the specific needs of each individual is essential.

In summary, the anti-inflammatory diet can offer significant benefits in cancer prevention and managing nutrition during therapies. It can help reduce inflammation in the body, provide nutritional support, and improve overall quality of life. However, it's important to remember that the diet does not replace traditional medicine and should always be integrated into a holistic and personalized approach to health.

Starting a new journey can seem like a daunting task, especially when it involves changing long-established habits. The approach we're about to describe is designed to make the transition as smooth as possible. It's not about revolutionizing everything at once but about taking small, progressive steps towards overall well-being.

First of all, let's get familiar with the concept of 'substitution'. We're not looking to drastically eliminate the foods we love, but to find healthier alternatives that are just as tasty. For example, if you love sweets, you might consider using natural sweeteners like honey or stevia instead of refined sugar. Similarly, if you're a fan of red meat, you might try to replace it more often with omega-3-rich fish or plant proteins such as legumes and tofu.

Another key strategy is increasing your intake of fruits and vegetables. Rich in fiber, antioxidants, and phytonutrients, these foods are real treasures for our bodies. Try to include at least one serving of fruit or vegetables at every meal. You can start with small changes, like adding a salad to your lunch or an apple as an afternoon snack.

Don't forget that water also plays a crucial role in this journey. Often, we forget to drink enough throughout the day, but water is essential for keeping our body hydrated and for promoting optimal functionality. Try to always carry a water bottle with you and create a habit of drinking regularly.

Remember, every person is unique. What works for someone might not work for you, and vice versa. Take time to listen to your body and observe how it reacts to these new habits. Be patient with yourself and celebrate every small success along the way.

This transition isn't a path to walk alone. Involve your loved ones, share your discoveries with them, and you can support each other in this extraordinary adventure towards more complete well-being. The journey of a thousand miles always begins with a single step.

An anti-inflammatory diet may be beneficial for a variety of conditions related to inflammation and immune system disorders. Here are some examples of conditions that may benefit from this type of diet:

Cancer: Some studies suggest that an anti-inflammatory diet can help reduce the inflammation that might promote cancer progression.

Rheumatoid arthritis: An autoimmune disease that causes chronic joint inflammation. An anti-inflammatory diet can help reduce symptoms and associated pain.

Autoimmune thyroid diseases, such as Hashimoto's thyroiditis: Reducing inflammation through diet may help manage symptoms and potentially moderate autoimmune activity.

Headaches, including chronic migraines: Inflammation can contribute to the frequency and intensity of headaches.

Gastritis: Inflammation of the stomach lining, which can be alleviated by reducing irritating and inflammatory foods.

Irritable Bowel Syndrome (IBS): An anti-inflammatory diet can help reduce gastrointestinal symptoms such as abdominal pain and bloating.

Heart disease: Inflammation is a known factor in the development of heart disease, and an anti-inflammatory diet can help reduce the risk.

Type 2 diabetes: Chronic inflammation is a significant risk factor for the development of diabetes, and diet can play a crucial role in controlling systemic inflammation.

Psoriasis: An autoimmune disease that affects the skin, causing redness and scaling.

Candidiasis: An overgrowth of Candida, a type of yeast, that can cause inflammation in various parts of the body, such as the mouth and intestines.

Adopting a diet rich in anti-inflammatory foods like fruits, vegetables, healthy fats, and lean proteins can help manage or improve these conditions.

Quote: *"Energy and persistence conquer all things." - Benjamin Franklin*

CHAPTER 2

"Brilliant Metabolism: Reactivate Your Energy and Well-being"

Your body is an incredible engineering system, and a fundamental part of this fascinating machine is the metabolism. But what exactly is metabolism? In simple terms, it's your body's internal engine that transforms food nutrients into energy. It's responsible for managing the energy your body needs to carry out every single activity, from the most complex to the most mundane.

The energy your body requires is produced through two main processes, known as basal metabolism and active metabolism. Basal metabolism is the energy your body uses for basic functions, such as breathing, making your heart beat, or maintaining body temperature, even when you're at rest. Active metabolism, on the other hand, is the energy your body uses for all other activities, such as running, jumping, thinking, speaking, and even reading this book.

But metabolism is much more than just an engine. It's also a delicate balance, a well-choreographed dance among your body's various processes. When this balance is disrupted, it can lead to health issues such as weight gain, fatigue, depression, and even more serious diseases. That's why it's so important to keep your metabolism in optimal shape.

Just as a car requires high-quality fuel to function at its best, the same is true for your body. The food you eat has a direct impact on your metabolism. Foods high in refined sugars and saturated fats can slow down your metabolism, while foods rich in proteins, fibers, and healthy fats can help keep it active and efficient.

But that's not all. Physical exercise also plays a crucial role in keeping your metabolism active. Physical activity helps build muscle mass, and the more muscle you have, the more calories your body burns, even at rest.

Your metabolism is a key element of your well-being. By keeping it active and efficient, you'll not only feel more energetic and vital, but you'll also be better able to manage your weight and prevent many diseases. And remember, every little choice counts. Every apple you choose instead of a donut, every time you opt to take the stairs instead of the elevator, you're doing something good for your metabolism. And your body will thank you.

The magic of living is not just in the breaths we take but also in the foods we consume. The decisions we make at the table are not matters of preference or routine, but significant milestones that define the course of our health. The anti-inflammatory diet emerges as a beacon in this vast dietary plain, guiding us toward nutritional choices that underscore our vitality, rather than undermine it.

Every bite of a carefully selected meal is an investment in your well-being. Anti-inflammatory foods like leafy greens, berries, nuts, seeds, omega-3-rich fish, and high-quality oils are packed with nutrients that work in tandem with your body, supporting efficient metabolic function.

Conversely, introducing inflammatory foods into your system can create barriers to its proper functioning. Foods high in refined sugars and trans fats can undermine your ability to efficiently convert food into energy.

With your willpower, you can direct this mechanism, making conscious choices that encourage energy and vitality, rather than hinder them. This is the power of an anti-inflammatory diet.

It's not just about weight loss or blood sugar control. This is a revolution in your relationship with food, embracing it as a powerful catalyst for well-being.

By adopting an anti-inflammatory diet, you're doing much more than revolutionizing your menu. You're reorganizing your internal biology, optimizing your metabolism to live with more energy and well-being. You're taking the reins, choosing a path that promotes your long-term health.

Food is much more than just a meal. It's a message to our body, a key to unlocking the full potential of our organism. And the anti-inflammatory diet is the interpreter that translates this message into a language our body can understand and use.

The adventure towards a brilliant metabolism starts with a single plate. A plate full of colors, flavors, and nutrients that promote our health.

There's something undeniably poetic about the rhythm of life—the rise and fall of the sun, the changing seasons, the rhythm of our breath. Yet, we tend to forget that our body has its rhythms too, regulated by our internal biological clock, also known as the "circadian rhythm." Among many functions, this rhythm regulates when we feel hungry and when we feel satiated. Ignoring these signals can disorient our body, throwing off the mechanisms that manage energy and satiety.

Meal timing is not just a matter of convenience. It's about aligning our eating rhythms with our body's rhythms, coordinating fuel with the machine. The right timing can make the difference between an efficient organism and one that struggles to keep up.

Start your day with a nutritious breakfast. We're not talking about a rushed cup of coffee or a cookie on the go. Take the time to nourish your body with proteins, fibers, and healthy fats to gently wake up your metabolism and provide the energy needed to start the day.

Make smart snacking choices between meals. This doesn't mean indulging in a bag of chips every time you feel a little hungry. Opt for nutrient-rich snacks that keep your blood sugar stable and prevent hunger pangs. A handful of nuts, a piece of fruit, a slice of whole-grain bread with avocado, are all valid options.

For lunch and dinner, choose balanced dishes with a good portion of proteins, healthy fats, and complex carbohydrates. This will help you feel satiated and provide the necessary energy for the rest of the day.

And perhaps most importantly, listen to your body. If you're not hungry, don't eat just because it's "mealtime". Similarly, don't ignore hunger just because it's not yet "mealtime". Your body is the best indicator of when it needs fuel.

Remember, food is a gift. It's a means to nourish both our body and soul. So, it's not just about "what" we eat, but also about "when" we eat it. Meal timing is a key ingredient in reactivating your energy and well-being. How about trying to dance to this rhythm?

Think of owning a beautiful, gleaming racehorse. A champion of strength and endurance, built to run. Now imagine keeping it tied up in a field all day, every day. No matter how much excellent grass you feed it, the horse will never reach its full potential unless it's allowed to run. This image reflects very clearly the interaction between our diet and physical exercise. You can provide your body with the best nutrition possible, but without physical activity, your body - like the horse - will not have the opportunity to fully express itself.

I'm not suggesting you need to become a marathon runner or a bodybuilder. Physical exercise doesn't have to be torture or a burdensome task. On the contrary, it should be something you enjoy, an activity that makes you feel alive and vigorous. It could be a brisk walk in the park, a yoga class, or a relaxing swim. The important thing is to move regularly and do something that you enjoy.

Regular physical activity has numerous benefits. Firstly, it increases the rate at which your body uses energy, improving your weight management ability. Secondly, it increases insulin sensitivity, helping to prevent blood sugar spikes that can cause fatigue and hunger. Moreover, physical exercise stimulates the production of endorphins, natural brain chemicals that enhance mood and overall well-being.

But perhaps most importantly, regular physical activity can help reduce stress levels, one of the main culprits behind many health problems. Our body reacts to stress by releasing hormones that can cause an increase in blood pressure, sleep disturbances, and a host of other health issues. Exercise helps to neutralize these effects, promoting deep relaxation and a sense of well-being.

In summary, physical exercise is a key component for optimizing body function and enhancing the effectiveness of a healthy diet. It's not just about burning calories, but about creating a more resilient, flexible, and capable body to face life's challenges. And remember, every movement counts. So, if you've never exercised before, start with small changes, and you'll see your body thank you. How about taking a small step today for your well-being?

What's your favorite superpower? Flying? Invisibility? How about an unstoppable immune system? Well, that's a capability you, the reader, already possess. Let me guide you in discovering how to fully leverage this powerful internal ally.

Our health is like a brick wall: sturdy and resilient, but each brick needs the others to keep the whole structure stable. The immune system is an essential brick in this wall, and its role in our health and wellbeing is of paramount importance. It's tasked with protecting us from external threats, like viruses and bacteria, and maintaining our internal processes in balance.

A strong immune system can be our best shield against many common diseases and conditions. Not only can it help us avoid colds and flu, but it can also protect us from more serious conditions. It's a tireless guardian working 24/7 to keep our body in balance.

But how can we fuel this superpower? First and foremost, healthy eating plays a critical role. A diet rich in fruits, vegetables, and whole foods provides our immune system with the vitamins and minerals it needs to function at its best. Additionally, exercise, as discussed earlier, improves circulation, facilitating the work of the immune system.

Another crucial aspect is rest. During sleep, our body has the chance to repair and regenerate itself, preparing for another day. Inadequate sleep can weaken the immune system, making us more susceptible to infections.

Prevention is much more effective than cure. Like a skilled sculptor, you can shape your health and well-being through your daily choices. And while we can't completely avoid diseases, a strong and responsive immune system can help us navigate these challenges more smoothly.

Consider prevention as an investment in your future. A small action today, like eating an extra piece of fruit or taking a daily walk, can have a significant impact on your long-term health. And remember, you're never alone on this journey. You, your body, and your powerful immune system are a team. So, ready to unleash your inner superpower?

Quote: *"The greatest wealth is health." - Virgil*

CHAPTER 3

"Guardians of the Body: Strengthening the Immune System for a Resilient Life"

Enter your personal armory: an invisible arsenal of defense, yet no less fascinating. It's your immune system, an internal network of guardians dedicated to maintaining the integrity and health of your body. Imagine being able to observe through a microscope this army of invisible cells at work.

An overview of this internal universe would first reveal two main actors. Antibodies, recognizable as tiny Ys floating in the bloodstream, are sent out to identify enemies: viruses, bacteria, anything that doesn't belong to your body. These tiny detectives are produced by B lymphocytes, which function a bit like a library of immune memories, storing information on every threat encountered.

But the keystone of this defense mechanism is the T lymphocytes, your front-line soldiers. When antibodies signal an intruder, T lymphocytes spring into action. Some of them attack the enemy directly, others send signals to recruit additional immune forces. And, in an act of your body's remarkable intelligence, some T lymphocytes "remember" the intruders, preparing your immune system for future similar challenges.

But how do we support these invisible troops? The answer is simple yet profound: by providing the right conditions for their success. Imagine training an army. Would you do it in an environment of chaos and scarcity? Or would you rather provide abundant resources, a clear strategy, and a favorable environment? The answer is obvious. And your immune system is no different.

A nutritious diet, physical exercise, adequate rest, stress management, and ultimately, love and joy, are all essential elements for creating optimal conditions for your immune system. These aren't just health clichés, but rather the pillars upon which the well-being of your entire body rests.

Herein lies the magic of your immune system: it is as invisible as it is essential. It's a silent witness to the challenges your body faces every day, responding with strength and adaptability. And with the right care, it can become an irreplaceable ally in your quest for a healthy and resilient life. So, are you ready to embrace your inner general and strengthen your internal army?

Our daily life is a journey, and the food we choose to consume is like the compass guiding us along the road. In this scenario, the anti-inflammatory diet is a golden compass, a sophisticated navigator steering us towards optimal health, helping us to nourish our immune system in the most comprehensive way possible.

In this ultra-connected world, we are flooded with information on what we should eat to achieve physical and mental well-being. Often, this information is distilled into a set of hard and fast rules, giving us the illusion that diet is merely a matter of mathematical calculations or adherence to a rigid plan. But friends, the truth is much more fascinating and nuanced.

Food is much more than mere fuel. It's the language our body uses to communicate with the outside world, a code that deciphers our relationship with the environment. When we consume nutrient-rich foods, we provide our immune system with the words that allow it to express itself at its best, to build a harmonious dialogue with its multiple functions.

Conversely, ultra-processed foods, filled with artificial additives, disrupt this delicate conversation. They are like background noise overshadowing our internal melody, leading our immune system to react instead of listen, to fight instead of cooperating. This can cause stress to our body, reducing its capacity to defend against diseases and infections.

This is where the anti-inflammatory diet comes into play, acting as a maestro orchestrating all the instruments of our internal symphony, allowing them to play together in perfect harmony. Natural and whole foods, rich in vitamins, minerals, and antioxidants, provide the notes our immune system needs to create its music, to build a balanced and constructive dialogue with its various parts.

Consider garlic and onions, with their potent antimicrobial properties, playing like a vigorous drum, strong and clear. Or kefir and other fermented foods, which support the health of the gut microbiota, adding a delicate touch, like a flute dancing lightly among deeper notes.

On this road to optimal health, the anti-inflammatory diet is our precious ally, our stellar navigator. It's not a magic solution but a journey of awareness and self-care, a way to honor our body and its incredible work. Because, when we nourish ourselves with attention and love, we're not just eating. We're building our internal symphony, creating our very own concert of health and well-being.

Peering into the world of vitamins and nutrients is like opening a box of colored gems, each with its uniqueness and distinctive value. These hidden treasures in our food play crucial roles in bolstering our immune resistance, equipping our body with the necessary tools to fend off harmful invaders.

Let's start with the **Vitamins**:

We welcome **Vitamin A**, an essential nutrient for eye health, body growth and development, and immune function. Vitamin A is found in foods like carrots, sweet potatoes, and kale.

Continuing our journey through the rich nutritional landscape, we encounter the **Vitamin B** complex. This team of vitamins, which includes B1, B2, B3, B5, B6, B7, B9, and B12, is vital for converting food into energy, keeping the nervous system functioning at its best, and contributing to the formation of red blood cells. You'll find these precious vitamins in a range of foods, including whole grains, potatoes, bananas, and legumes.

Let's not forget **Vitamin C**, a little hero with big actions. Sometimes underestimated, it's a powerful antioxidant that strengthens white blood cells, the frontline soldiers in the fight against infections and diseases. Nothing beats a juicy citrus fruit or fresh strawberries to load up on this essential vitamin.

Then there's **Vitamin D**, the miniature sun of our organism. A deficiency in vitamin D can weaken our immune system, but fortunately, it's abundantly available through sunlight exposure. Adding foods like salmon or eggs to our diet can provide an extra boost to our vitamin D levels.

Vitamin E, the guardian of our cellular health. This fat-soluble vitamin is a powerful antioxidant that protects our cells from oxidative stress. It's like a personal bodyguard for every single cell in our body. We can find it in foods like nuts, seeds, and olive oil.

Vitamin K is a vital nutrient for blood clotting and maintaining strong bones. Leafy green vegetables like spinach, kale, and lettuce are excellent sources of vitamin K.

Let's talk about **Minerals**:

We meet **Potassium**, a mineral that helps regulate blood pressure, reduces water retention, and protects against strokes. It's essential for the proper functioning of nerves and muscles, including those of the heart. Potassium is abundant in fruits and vegetables like bananas, oranges, and spinach.

Magnesium often overlooked but of fundamental importance. Magnesium supports hundreds of enzyme reactions in our body, including those involving the immune system's function. Rich in foods like leafy green vegetables and legumes, each serving of these foods provides additional armor to our immune system.

Let's not forget about **Iron**, a key component of hemoglobin that helps white blood cells function at their best. Iron is present in many foods, including red meat, lentils, and spinach. Each bite of these foods provides a boost of strength to our immune system.

Zinc, a nutrient that often goes unnoticed but is crucial for the immune system's functioning. Zinc is a great ally, contributing to wound healing and fighting off viruses. It's abundant in foods like oysters, beef, and pumpkin seeds.

We can't overlook **Calcium**, an essential mineral for the health of bones and teeth, but also for muscle and nerve function. Calcium is plentiful in foods like milk, yogurt, cheese, and leafy green vegetables.

We also meet **Phosphorus**. This mineral not only helps build strong bones and teeth but is also indispensable for the production of proteins necessary for the growth, maintenance, and repair of body cells and tissues. Foods like dairy products, meat, and fish are rich in phosphorus.

Copper is another essential element. This trace mineral helps produce red blood cells, responsible for transporting oxygen to the body's tissues. Foods-like liver, oysters, nuts, and sunflower seeds are good sources of copper.

Selenium, another trace mineral, is crucial for regulating metabolism and for the proper functioning of the thyroid. Furthermore, selenium is known for its antioxidant properties. Foods like tuna, Brazil nuts, sunflower seeds, and chicken are rich in selenium.

The picture that emerges is that of a complex mosaic of nutrients working together to create a masterpiece - a resilient immune system. The next time you sit down for a meal, think about the vitamins and minerals you're about to ingest. Every bite is a brick contributing to building your immune defense, a step forward towards optimal health. It's not just what you eat, but how you eat it. With pleasure, with appreciation, and above all, with awareness.

There are many aspects of our lifestyle that can directly impact the robustness of our immune system. It's not just what we eat, but also how we live that can have a significant impact on our health and disease resistance. Sleep, physical exercise, and stress, as we've also reiterated in previous chapters, are just some of the factors that can alter the ability of our immune system to do its job properly.

Let's start with Sleep. If we think of sleep as a kind of nightly maintenance for our body, its importance becomes clear. During sleep, our body works to repair and regenerate cells, as well as to strengthen our memory and cognitive functions. Insufficient or poor-quality sleep can make our immune system less responsive, leaving us more vulnerable to illnesses.

Now let's move on to Physical Exercise. Regular physical activity not only keeps our body in shape but also has a stimulating effect on our immune system. Exercise helps improve circulation, allowing immune system cells and substances to move freely in the body and do their job more efficiently.

Stress, on the other hand, is a factor that can put a strain on our immune system. Prolonged stress situations can indeed alter the balance of our body, negatively affecting the immune system and increasing our susceptibility to diseases.

Managing stress through techniques such as meditation, yoga, or simply dedicating time to activities we love, can have a positive effect on our immune health.

Taking care of our lifestyle is just as important as paying attention to what we eat. Good sleep, regular exercise, and effective stress management are essential to keep our immune system strong and resilient. Finding the right balance isn't always easy, but small changes can lead to significant benefits. Your body is a wonderfully complex and resilient system that deserves your care and attention.

Our health, including that of our immune system, doesn't just depend on us alone but is intrinsically connected to the world around us. The environment we live in, and our social relationships can directly and indirectly influence our immune health.

First, let's consider the environment. We live in an increasingly urbanized world, where air and noise pollution have become constant concerns. These elements can cause stress and lead to conditions that compromise our immune health. It's not just about avoiding these harmful situations but about creating positive environments. Green spaces, clean air, and a peaceful environment can help reduce stress and improve overall health, including the immune system.

Regarding social relationships, their importance for our health cannot be overstated. Positive relationships can act as a buffer against stress and provide support in times of need. Conversely, tense, or conflictual relationships can cause chronic stress, which can compromise our immune health. Therefore, cultivating positive relationships and building a strong support network is crucial.

The act of helping others can also have a positive impact on our health. Volunteering, caring for others, and donating to those less fortunate can create a sense of well-being and happiness, which in turn can strengthen our immune system.

To maintain a strong immune system, we must not only look after ourselves but also the environment around us and the people we interact with. Creating a healthy environment and cultivating positive relationships can have a profound effect on our immune health. Remember, we are social creatures and part of a larger ecosystem. Our health reflects this fact, so let's take care not only of ourselves but also of the world around us.

Prevention is a word we should keep in mind when thinking about our health. It's so easy to fall into the trap of reacting to health problems only when they arise. But the real key to long-term health and longevity is prevention, and our immune system plays a vital role in this process.

A robust immune system is not just a defender against diseases; it's the guardian of our health, constantly working to neutralize potential threats before they can cause harm. It's our first and most important bastion against a vast number of diseases and conditions.

From this perspective, preventing rather than curing means not just avoiding risky behaviors or following an exercise regime. It also means taking care of our immune system by nourishing it with a healthy diet, ensuring adequate rest, reducing stress, and maintaining strong social bonds.

We should remember that our immune system doesn't act alone. It's inextricably linked to our body and our mind. Anxiety and stress can compromise its effectiveness, as can a diet lacking in essential nutrients. On the other hand, a calm mind, a well-rested body, and a balanced diet can provide the support it needs to function at its best.

Prevention is not a one-time action but a continuous process. It's a commitment we make to ourselves to live life in the healthiest way possible. We shouldn't wait to get sick before we start taking our health seriously. We need to make daily choices that support our immune system and, ultimately, our overall health.

So, dear Reader, let's always remember prevention is better than cure. And one of the best forms of prevention is maintaining a strong and healthy immune system. Health is a precious treasure. Let's take care of this treasure, not only for ourselves but also for the people we love. Our health is not just in the hands of doctors or medicines, but is also, and most importantly, in our own hands.

Quote: *"Food: our body is its mirror." - Hippocrates*

CHAPTER 4

"The Power on the Plate: Inflammatory vs. Anti-inflammatory Foods"

The term "inflammation" might seem alien and distant from our everyday lives. Yet, it's closer than we think. Our body uses inflammation as an alarm signal, a bell that rings when something is wrong. But when this defense mechanism malfunctions, it becomes an issue that can lead to diseases like diabetes, obesity, and heart problems. In this scenario, what we put on our plate becomes the conductor of this delicate balance.

Diabetes, for example, is not just a matter of sugars. Behind the scenes, chronic inflammation can play a key role in sabotaging the body's ability to use insulin properly, the hormone that helps us manage blood sugar levels. When we consume foods that promote inflammation, we are essentially giving free rein to this internal sabotage.

Similarly, obesity is not just a matter of calories. Beneath the surface, chronic inflammation can alter the way the body handles calories and weight. Certain foods, such as those high in refined sugars and saturated fats, can kickstart a cycle of inflammation and fat accumulation, making weight loss an uphill battle.

Regarding heart problems, inflammation can be a silent but powerful factor. Chronic inflammation can damage blood vessels and promote plaque buildup, which in turn can increase the risk of diseases like arteriosclerosis, hypertension, and heart attack.

The good news is that we are not powerless in the face of all this. While some foods can promote inflammation, others can help us fight it. By choosing foods rich in antioxidants, fiber, and healthy fats, we can help maintain our body's balance and defend ourselves from these diseases.

It's not just about food, but about choices, awareness, and the power we have over ourselves. The power to choose what to put on our plate and to determine the course of our health. It's a story that each of us writes day by day, a story about health and life. And this is a story that deserves to be told.

Exploring the universe of foods can be an adventure full of discoveries, but also surprises. Some foods that seem harmless or even healthy can actually do more harm than good, especially when it comes to inflammation.

Let's start with foods high in **Refined Sugars**: Think of cookies, cakes, and sugary drinks. Yes, they can offer moments of sweetness, but at a high price. These foods cause spikes in blood sugar that put the body in an alert state, as if it were under attack. The response is inflammation. In the long term, this can lead to problems such as insulin resistance, the cornerstone of type 2 diabetes.

Fried Foods: While the occasional fried potato or fried chicken might seem harmless, fried foods contain high amounts of trans fats and omega-6 fatty acids, which can promote inflammation. Moreover, the frying process can produce toxic compounds like acrylamide, which can contribute to chronic inflammation and increase the risk of diseases.

Gluten is another protagonist: Found in many grains like wheat, barley, and rye, it can be problematic for those with celiac disease or gluten sensitivity. In these cases, gluten can trigger an immune reaction that causes inflammation and damage to the intestine.

Dairy: Can be an issue for those who are intolerant or allergic. In these individuals, the consumption of dairy products can cause symptoms like bloating, abdominal pain, and diarrhea, signs of ongoing inflammation.

Processed Red Meat: While unprocessed red meat can be part of a healthy diet, obviously always in the right limits, processed meat like sausages, hams, bacon, hot dogs, and other processed meats can contain preservatives like nitrates and nitrites, which can promote inflammation. These foods often also contain high amounts of salt and saturated fats, both known for their ability to promote inflammation. They can increase blood pressure and the risk of cardiovascular diseases.

Energy Drinks: These beverages often contain high levels of sugars and caffeine. Excessive consumption of sugars, as we've seen, can lead to blood glucose spikes that promote inflammation. Additionally, caffeine in large quantities can cause elevated blood pressure and hormonal stress, which can, in turn, trigger inflammation.

Alcohol: Alcohol consumption can be a double blow to our body. It can lead to increased inflammation in the liver and damage it.

Sugary Drinks: Sugary drinks, like soft drinks, are filled with simple sugars. Regular consumption of these beverages can lead to an increase in body weight, insulin resistance, and inflammation. These effects can be particularly harmful to the heart and can increase the risk of cardiovascular diseases.

Now, it's not about demonizing these foods or completely eliminating everything from our plate. It's about understanding how food affects our body and making informed choices. Sometimes, careful moderation can make the difference between a body in balance and one in conflict with itself. And in this choice lies an important part of our health and well-being. Let's always remember that knowledge is power, and on our plate lies a power that can shape our well-being and health.

Transitioning from the minefield of unhealthy food choices to the serenity of a well-balanced diet doesn't have to be an insurmountable climb. This is precisely where anti-inflammatory foods come into play, a team of nutritional superheroes ready to defend us, strengthen our health, and prevent diseases.

One of the key players in this team is **Fish**, known for its high content of omega-3 fatty acids. These nutrients are essential in reducing inflammation, preventing the formation of plaques in the arteries, and lowering blood pressure. Furthermore, the benefits of an omega-3-rich diet can extend to the brain, supporting memory and cognition.

Speaking of fish, we cannot overlook Salmon, Sardines, and Cod. These fish are rich sources of omega-3 fatty acids and are well-known for their anti-inflammatory properties. Moreover, fish oil has been shown to help reduce inflammation and can have beneficial effects on heart health.

The **Seafood** world offers numerous options that can make a difference in an anti-inflammatory diet. Mussels, for example, can be a brilliant choice. These shellfish are loaded with omega-3 fatty acids and essential minerals like zinc, which strengthen our immune system and help reduce inflammation.

Another beneficial seafood is Clams, which not only offer a good dose of omega-3 but are also among the best sources of iron, an essential nutrient for maintaining energy and overall health.

Moving to the realm of **White Meats**, Chicken is a popular and versatile option. However, it's important to be mindful of the source of this meat: opting for organic, free-range chicken can make a significant difference in nutritional quality. Chicken is a lean source of protein, necessary for repairing body tissues and reducing inflammation. Another anti inflammatory ally in the world of white meats is turkey, an excellent source of lean protein and tryptophan, an amino acid that can help improve mood and sleep quality, two key aspects in combating chronic inflammation.

Fruit, with its splendid hues and natural sweetness, is not just a delight for the palate but also a boon for our health. Consider Blueberries and Cherries, whose antioxidant properties are well known. But also, Pineapple and Papaya, rich in enzymes like bromelain and papain, which have anti-inflammatory actions.

In the exuberant landscape of fruits, two more notable allies are Plums and Apples. Plums, with their rich content of vitamin C and potassium, are a great resource for cardiovascular health, supporting normal blood pressure and fighting inflammation. Apples, in addition to being an important source of dietary fiber for gut health, contain a variety of phytonutrients that perform antioxidant and anti-inflammatory functions, offering a significant contribution to overall well-being. Each fruit, with its unique properties, is a small jewel of nourishment for our body.

Avocado, rich in heart-healthy monounsaturated fats, helps to lower levels of bad cholesterol in the blood and improve nutrient absorption. Additionally, it contains carotenoids, vitamins C and E, which have antioxidant and anti-inflammatory properties.

Then, there are our colorful friends, the **Berries**. Rich in antioxidants and phytonutrients, these little health gems work to neutralize free radicals, protecting cells from oxidative damage. They are also excellent for heart health and can help regulate blood sugar levels.

In the varied universe of **Vegetables**, we can find true warriors for our well-being. Take, for example, Carrots and Squash, which, with their high content of vitamin A, play a key role in keeping our immune system balanced. Let's not forget Beetroot, with its rich assortment of antioxidants like betalain, which has been shown to have effective anti-inflammatory properties. Vegetables represent a valuable ally on our journey towards optimal health, offering a set of vital nutrients.

Kale, for instance, thanks to its abundance of vitamin K, helps to maintain the balance of our immune system.

Spinach these leafy green vegetables are rich in vitamins, minerals, and phytonutrients, including carotenoids, vitamin C, vitamin K, folic acid, and calcium. Their antioxidant and anti-inflammatory properties help protect the body's cells from oxidative damage.

Broccoli, known for its anti-cancer properties, also contains a compound called sulforaphane, known for its anti-inflammatory properties. This healthy vegetable is also a great source of vitamins K and C, as well as fiber, folate, and potassium.

Bell Peppers are rich in vitamin C and various carotenoids, which have powerful antioxidant and anti-inflammatory properties. They help protect the skin from sun damage, promote eye health, and may reduce the risk of some chronic diseases.

Tomatoes are rich in lycopene, a carotenoid that has been shown to have strong anti-inflammatory properties. Lycopene is particularly effective in reducing inflammation in the lungs and throughout the body. Additionally, tomatoes are a great source of vitamin C and potassium.

Let's not forget **Nuts and Seeds**. Almonds, Walnuts, and Flaxseeds are all foods we should try to include in our diet. Besides being rich in omega-3 fatty acids, they also contain other antioxidant and anti-inflammatory substances like vitamin E.

Walnuts are also a great source of healthy fats, including omega-3 fatty acids. They help reduce inflammation, improve heart health, and can help protect the brain.

Grains, essential in a balanced diet, can do their part in fighting inflammation. Spelt, for example, with its generous dose of fiber, helps regulate digestion and reduce inflammation. Oats, rich in beta-glucans, help keep blood cholesterol levels low, promoting heart health. Finally, Millet, a gluten-free grain, contains magnesium and coenzyme Q10, essential elements for cellular health.

Legumes, in turn, are a treasure trove of beneficial nutrients. Lentils, for example, provide a good dose of fiber, protein, and minerals, helping to maintain the balance of the gut microbiota and reduce inflammation. Chickpeas, rich in protein and fiber, can help regulate blood sugar levels and reduce inflammation. Black beans, with their high antioxidant content, can help counteract the damaging action of free radicals.

Let's also talk about **Yogurt**, which deserves a place of honor among anti-inflammatory foods. This fermented dairy product is a valuable source of probiotics, the so-called "good bacteria," that help maintain the health of our intestinal flora. A balanced gut microbiota is crucial for preventing systemic inflammation. Additionally, rich in proteins and calcium, it provides essential nutrients for muscle and bone health. To enjoy all its benefits, it's best to choose natural yogurt, without added sugars or artificial flavors. Greek yogurt, in particular, is known for its high protein content and creaminess. You can sweeten it with a bit of honey for a dessert or snack that's both delicious and good for your body.

Another unexpected helper in the fight against inflammation is **Extra Virgin Olive Oil**. Oleocanthal, a compound found in it, has anti-inflammatory effects that can be comparable to those of over-the-counter medications, with the advantage of not having side effects.

And let's not forget about **Spices** like Turmeric and Ginger. Turmeric contains curcumin, which has potent anti-inflammatory and antioxidant effects. Ginger, with its gingerol, is known for reducing inflammation and promoting digestion.

Green Tea is another healthy ally. With its generous dose of epigallocatechin gallate (EGCG), a potent antioxidant, green tea can help reduce the risk of heart disease, improve brain function, and aid in weight management.

And finally, the **Honey**. This precious gift from bees is not just sweet to the taste but also a sweet benefit to health. Honey contains flavonoids and polyphenols, potent antioxidants that fight inflammation. Moreover, some honeys, like manuka honey, are known for their antibacterial and anti-inflammatory properties.

When we talk about food, it's common to imagine delicious dishes that delight the palate. However, on a deeper level, foods are genuine chemical laboratories that significantly influence our health.

Consider, for example, antioxidants. These little warriors are natural chemicals found in many of the foods we've already mentioned, such as fruits, vegetables, and whole grains. Their main job? To protect our cells from damage caused by free radicals, unstable molecules that can cause inflammation and accelerate cellular aging. Antioxidants act as shields, neutralizing free radicals before they can cause harm.

But there's more. In addition to antioxidants, many foods are rich in phytonutrients, chemicals produced by plants that offer numerous health benefits. Phytonutrients can play a crucial role in keeping inflammation levels low, boosting the immune system, protecting the heart, and much more. What's truly interesting is that these phytonutrients often give foods their characteristic color: lycopene in red tomatoes, for example, or anthocyanins in blue and purple berries.

Finally, let's talk about Omega-3 fatty acids. These polyunsaturated fatty acids, found in foods like fatty fish, flaxseeds, and walnuts, are powerful allies in the fight against inflammation. They act by interfering with the production of chemicals that promote inflammation, thus helping to maintain our body's balance.

Reflect for a moment on this information. Every time we eat, we're not just satisfying our hunger. We're providing our body with the chemical tools it needs to fight inflammation, protect our cells, and maintain our health. The plate of colorful vegetables we're about to consume isn't just a feast for the eyes and palate but a true health cocktail.

The chemistry of food isn't an abstract concept or far from our daily lives. It's a reality we live at every meal, a dance of molecules that silently helps us build our well-being. Eating thus becomes not just a pleasure but also a conscious act and a gift to our health.

Carotenoids are plant pigments responsible for the yellow, orange, and red hues of many fruits and vegetables. Among the most well-known is beta-carotene, found abundantly in carrots, which our body can convert into vitamin A, essential for eye health and the immune system. But carotenoids aren't just "natural colorings": they also play an important role in protecting our body from inflammation and damage from free radicals.

Glucosinolates are sulfur-containing compounds that give cruciferous vegetables, like broccoli and Brussels sprouts, their characteristic slightly bitter and pungent flavor. These phytonutrients have been studied for their powerful anti-inflammatory and anti-cancer properties. In fact, once ingested, glucosinolates are transformed by our body into bioactive molecules that can neutralize carcinogens and reduce inflammation.

Here, then, are two more silent heroes hidden in the colors and flavors of our foods, working tirelessly for our health.

Now, imagine embarking on a very special mission: entering a supermarket armed with insights and wise choices, aiming to leave with a cart full of allies for your health. Sounds like an adventure, right? Well, in reality, that's exactly what you're about to do. Through these strategies for smart shopping, you will be able to promote an anti-inflammatory diet.

First, it's important to have a plan. Before setting foot in the supermarket, prepare a list of the foods you need. Ensure that the list is full of fresh and nutritious foods, from seafood to seasonal vegetables, from whole grains to legumes, and minimize processed foods.

Speaking of processed foods, learn to read labels carefully. Often, processed foods contain added sugars, salt, and unhealthy fats, all factors that can fuel inflammation in the body. Don't be fooled by health claims printed on the package; what really matters are the ingredients.

Third, prioritize quality over quantity. A free-range chicken or a wild-caught fish may cost more, but they are also richer in beneficial nutrients and less likely to contain antibiotics or other additives that can fuel inflammation. The same goes for organic vegetables, which are grown without the use of chemical pesticides.

Fourth, bring home a variety of foods. Each food has a unique nutritional profile, so the more varied your diet, the broader the spectrum of nutrients you'll intake. Vary the colors of the foods you choose, too: the phytonutrients that give vegetables and fruits their color also has potent anti-inflammatory properties.

Consider shopping at local markets or farms. Not only will you have the opportunity to buy fresh and seasonal foods, but you'll also be supporting the local economy.

Now that you're armed with these strategies, you're ready to shop smartly. Remember, every choice you make can be a step toward better health.

Quote: *"Health is the real wealth, not pieces of gold and silver." - Gandhi*

CHAPTER 5

"Shape and Health: Losing Weight with Taste and Wisdom"

"Diet or Lifestyle?" Whenever we tackle the topic of weight, this question looms like a crossroads before us. Do we choose the path of dieting, with its frantic pace and ephemeral successes, or do we take the road of lifestyle, with its gradual but lasting changes? This choice might seem like a dilemma, but in reality, when examined closely, a surprisingly simple truth emerges.

The word diet immediately conjures up ideas of restriction, sacrifice, and, in many cases, the dreaded "yo-yo effect." Losing weight through dieting might seem like an immediate success, but it often leads to an equally rapid weight regain once old eating patterns resume.

On the other hand, adopting a new healthy lifestyle is a process that occurs calmly and consistently. It's a change that takes root deeply and alters not only our eating habits but also our view of food and wellness in general. It's not about deprivation, but about discovery. Discovering new flavors, new combinations, new dishes that nourish the body and satisfy the palate. This is why a lifestyle change is more likely to be sustainable in the long term: not because it's easy, but because it awakens a genuine pleasure in eating healthily.

A new lifestyle doesn't exclude weight loss but sees it as a positive side effect of healthier and more conscious choices. It's a transformation that starts with small steps, such as preferring whole grains over refined ones or increasing the intake of fruits and vegetables. But every small step, over time, can lead to surprising results.

The key, on this journey, is kindness towards oneself. Accepting that there will be highs and lows, that there will be days when it will be hard to resist temptation. But what really matters is not perfection but consistency. And with consistency and patience, that coveted balance between taste and wisdom can become an everyday reality.

So, "diet or lifestyle?" The answer is in your hands or, better, on your plate. And remember it's not about giving up the pleasure of eating, but about rediscovering it in a healthier and more sustainable form.

The road to weight loss should never be a path paved with deprivation, calorie counting, or exhausting workouts. It shouldn't be a journey tormented by rigid boundaries and constraints. Instead, imagine if your path to a lighter and healthier you were a journey of discovery, of connection with your body, of understanding what truly fuels and nourishes it. Herein lies the essence of the anti-inflammatory diet.

This is not a diet in the traditional sense of the term, not a temporary deprivation plan for quick, unsustainable weight loss. It's a way of living, a way of eating, which focuses on the nutrients that rebalance your body, calming inflammation, balancing your metabolism, freeing your body to do what it's designed to do: thrive.

When you introduce anti-inflammatory foods into your life—freely swimming fatty fish, wild berries, leafy green vegetables—you're not just introducing tasty dishes. You're triggering a gear shift in your body. You're taking control, telling your body that it's time to release the fat it has stored, to restore natural metabolic processes.

And what about the yo-yo effect, the return of lost pounds that often follows stricter diets? This is the beauty of the anti-inflammatory diet. It's not a "program to follow" that you then abandon. It's a journey you embark on, a way of living you embrace. It's not about restriction but liberation. You don't eliminate foods; you replace them. You discover new flavors, new pleasures, and, in this process, find a balance that works for you. It's a freedom that not only promotes weight loss but builds a future of well-being.

Losing weight won't feel like a struggle but like an adventure. It's not about being enslaved to the scale but about listening to your body. It's an invitation to become the custodian of your well-being, with the audacity to experiment, the curiosity to discover, and the determination to thrive. This is the true promise of the anti-inflammatory diet. It's more than a diet; it's a life change. And isn't that a wonderful journey to embark on?

Now, we encounter a concept often overlooked but of vital importance: listening to your body. This isn't just about recognizing the need for rest or movement but also interpreting its delicate cues about satiety.

We're often accustomed to eating according to set times and portions, ignoring the signals our body sends us. We've been conditioned to believe that we need to consume three meals a day, regardless of hunger, or that it's essential to clear the plate, despite feeling full. It's time to relearn to listen to our body, to understand when we're genuinely hungry and when we're satisfied.

Learning to recognize the feeling of satiety is a journey of self-discovery. You'll start to notice the difference between physical hunger and emotional hunger, understanding that eating isn't the only way to manage stress or boredom. This awareness is a powerful ally in portion control. It's not about drastically limiting quantities but about listening to your body and respecting its needs.

And this is where the art of mindful eating comes into play. It's not just about what we put on our plate, but how we do it. Eating slowly, savoring each bite, focusing on the food rather than the phone screen or television. This mindful attention not only increases the pleasure of eating but also allows your body to register satiety signals, preventing overeating.

The quality of the food you eat is crucial, but how you eat it is equally important. Listening to your body, respecting its needs, and consciously enjoying each bite: these are the tools that will allow you to manage portions without feeling deprived or hungry. They are the tools that will transform a meal into a moment of care, of connection with yourself.

It's not an easy path, but it's worth it. Because, when you start listening to your body, you begin to understand its needs, and this understanding is the key to optimal health and balanced weight. So, step by step, listen after listen, you'll discover that the road to well-being isn't a path paved with deprivation but a path of awareness, respect, and love for yourself.

Let's explore a new perspective on the concept of weight loss. We transform our vision, no longer focused on shrinking the numbers on the scale, but rather on building a body and mind in full health. Physical activity, in this scenario, becomes a fundamental component, not only for weight loss but for the overall well-being of the person.

The keyword here is "balance." To achieve a healthy weight and maintain it over time, it's essential to combine physical exercise with proper nutrition. This combination offers 360-degree benefits, going far beyond simple weight loss: it improves heart health, promotes quality sleep, helps reduce stress, and provides energy.

Physical exercise doesn't necessarily mean going to the gym or enduring grueling workouts. Instead, it's important to find an activity you truly love, something that becomes a pleasant appointment rather than an obligation. Consider running, for example, an activity that can be practiced anywhere, outdoors or on a treadmill, and offers great cardiovascular benefits.

Another valuable ally is yoga, a meeting of body and mind that improves flexibility, strengthens muscles, and promotes inner serenity. And what about swimming, a real boon for the whole body, or dancing, which allows you to burn calories while having fun and strengthens coordination and balance?

Furthermore, for those who prefer low-impact activities, walking is an excellent starting point. Every step, every breath, is an act of self-love, an opportunity to connect with one's body, to observe the world with new eyes.

Then there's cycling, perfect for toning the legs and enjoying the charm of outdoor movement. The important thing is to move, respecting your own rhythms and needs. Physical activity is not a punishment but an opportunity: the chance to take care of yourself, to feel your body live and vibrate with energy.

While a balanced diet is essential for weight loss, it's equally true that physical exercise is the perfect travel companion on this journey. The synergy between these two elements will lead to lasting results, a healthy body, and a calm mind. And in the end, that's what matters: feeling good about yourself, in full health and harmony with your body.

A world of colors, scents, and flavors. This is how the kaleidoscope of food temptations presents itself, ready to capture our attention in moments of weakness. But what if these temptations could become opportunities for growth? If they could teach us to know ourselves better, to discover the strength we have inside?

Let's start with a consideration: slip-ups are part of the journey. They are not failures but opportunities to learn. Every time we face an obstacle, we can choose to see it as an insurmountable wall or as a step that allows us to climb higher. Our attitude makes the difference.

Learning to manage food temptations is a process that requires time, patience, and a good dose of self-compassion. It's not about fighting against us but understanding our emotions, welcoming them, and guiding them. Here, coping strategies come into play, useful techniques for dealing with stress and keeping focus on our goals.

A first step might be to identify the triggers, i.e., those events or situations that lead us to eat impulsively. Once recognized, we can try to avoid these situations or prepare ourselves to manage them. For example, if we know that after a stressful day at work we tend to seek refuge in food, we could plan a relaxing activity when we get home, like a walk or a pilates session, or simply reading a book.

Another strategy is time management. Dividing the day into pleasant and satisfying activities can reduce the temptation to eat out of boredom or to fill a void. Let's remember to dedicate time to ourselves, our hobbies, and the people we love.

Finally, it's important to cultivate positive self-talk. Talk to ourselves as we would to a dear friend. Let's remember our successes, the steps we have already taken. If we let ourselves be discouraged by a small slip-up, we might lose sight of all the progress we've made.

In managing temptations, the most powerful weapon is awareness. The awareness of being human, with our strengths and weaknesses. The awareness that every day is a new opportunity to make choices that bring us closer to health and well-being. And above all, the awareness that we are the protagonists of our journey, and that we possess everything we need to navigate towards our goal.

Quote: *"Food can be the most powerful form of medicine or the slowest form of poison." - Ann Wigmore.*

CHAPTER 6

"Emotions and Body in Harmony: Physical and Emotional Effects of Diet"

Our diet goes beyond the mere necessity of nourishing the body. In an era where mental health is finally receiving the attention it deserves, it's worth exploring how our food choices can influence our psychological well-being.

Let's start with a simple example: when you're sad or stressed, what do you choose to eat? Maybe you find comfort in something sweet, or perhaps you lose your appetite altogether. In both cases, your emotions are guiding your food choices, and at the same time, what you eat affects your mood. It's an interconnected cycle, a delicate balance we often overlook.

We must acknowledge that it's not just about "comfort food." Science is discovering that what we eat can have a real and tangible impact on our mental health. For instance, a diet rich in fruits, vegetables, legumes, nuts, and seeds, combined with moderate consumption of fish, meat, and dairy, has been linked to a lower risk of depression. Conversely, diets high in sugar can increase the risk of depression and anxiety.

Think about what happens when you eat a balanced meal. Your blood sugar levels stabilize, avoiding spikes and drops that can affect your mood. By consuming proteins, you provide your body with the amino acids necessary to produce neurotransmitters like serotonin, often referred to as the "happiness hormone."

Serotonin is an important neurotransmitter for regulating mood, sleep, and appetite. It's not directly present in foods, but some contain tryptophan, an amino acid that the body can convert into serotonin. Here are some foods rich in tryptophan:

Eggs: Eggs are an excellent source of tryptophan, in addition to being rich in high-quality proteins and other beneficial nutrients.

Pumpkin Seeds: These seeds not only contain a large amount of tryptophan but also zinc, which helps convert tryptophan into serotonin.

Turkey: Like many other lean meats, turkey is a good source of tryptophan.

Salmon: Salmon is known for its richness in omega-3 fatty acids, but it's also a good source of tryptophan.

Spinach: Spinach contains a significant amount of tryptophan. It's also full of other essential nutrients, such as iron and vitamins A and C.

Milk: This food is a well-known source of tryptophan. Moreover, its soothing nature makes a warm cup of milk a popular choice for those who have trouble sleeping.

Coconut Oil: This oil, extracted from the flesh of coconuts, contains tryptophan. It's also rich in medium-chain fatty acids that can promote brain health.

Brazil Nuts: These nuts are known for their tryptophan content and are often consumed as a snack or incorporated into recipes to increase the intake of this essential amino acid.

Kiwi is a fruit rich in serotonin. Beyond its delicious taste, kiwi offers a wide range of health benefits thanks to its richness in vitamins and minerals. It's notably known for containing tryptophan, the amino acid that the body uses to produce serotonin, thus helping to promote balanced moods and restful sleep.

Brown Rice is another excellent source of tryptophan, the amino acid necessary for the production of serotonin. This makes brown rice a great food for promoting mental well-being. Consuming brown rice not only provides a steady supply of energy thanks to its richness in complex carbohydrates, but it also contributes to the production of serotonin, thus fostering a positive mood and quality sleep.

Cantaloupe, in particular, is another fantastic ally for our mental well-being. This tasty fruit is rich in vitamin B6, a vitamin that plays a key role in the production of serotonin in the brain. Additionally, cantaloupe also contains a good amount of vitamin C, a potent antioxidant that can help protect the brain from oxidative stress.

Consuming cantaloupe can not only boost serotonin production but also refresh us during hot summer days, offering a sweet and refreshing flavor that's hard to resist.

And it's not just serotonin. There are other neurotransmitters that depend on what we eat. For example, dopamine, which is involved in our brain's reward system, can be stimulated by certain foods.

Dopamine, another neurotransmitter, plays a crucial role in our brain's reward system, giving us a sense of pleasure and motivation. There are no foods that contain dopamine directly, but some can help the body produce it. Here are some examples:

Apples can contribute to dopamine production. This fruit contains high levels of antioxidants, which can help protect brain cells and support dopamine production. Additionally, apples contain vitamin C, known for its ability to increase dopamine levels.

Bananas, especially when ripe, are rich in tyrosine, an amino acid that the body converts into dopamine.

Avocado not only contains tyrosine but also healthy fats, fiber, and antioxidants.

Almonds are another source of tyrosine. They also contain a variety of essential nutrients, including fiber, vitamin E, and healthy fats.

Beans, especially black beans, are rich in tyrosine. Besides, they are an excellent source of fiber and protein.

Strawberries contain tyrosine and are also full of antioxidants and vitamin C.

Dark Chocolate is another food that can contribute to dopamine production. It's rich in antioxidants and can help stimulate the release of dopamine in the brain. It's important to remember it should be consumed in moderation due to its sugar content.

However, it's crucial to understand that this is not about replacing medical or psychological treatment with a diet. Instead, it's about complementing the care of our minds with the care of our bodies. Recognizing the link between diet and mental health is a fundamental step towards overall well-being.

Our dietary choices not only build our physique but also our mood, our ability to concentrate, our resilience to stress. And if this isn't a reason to pay more attention to what we put on our plate, then what else could be?

"Eating" is an act we perform multiple times a day, yet how often do we stop to truly think about what we're doing? How often do we eat distractedly, in a hurry, without even tasting what we're ingesting? The practice of **Mindful Eating** invites us to bring awareness back to the mealtime, creating a healthier and more balanced relationship with food.

Mindful Eating isn't a diet or a set of rules about what or how much to eat, but rather an approach to food that encourages full awareness of what you eat and why you eat. This means taking note of the colors, smells, flavors, and tastes of the food. It means paying attention to the sensations of hunger and satiety and recognizing the emotional responses we might have to food.

To start practicing Mindful Eating, we might get into the habit of sitting at the table without distractions, listening to our body. Instead of eating automatically, we ask ourselves: am I really hungry? Or am I eating because I'm stressed, bored, or sad? Opening the door to these questions begins to better understand our eating habits and the role food plays in our lives.

Another key aspect of Mindful Eating is the appreciation of food. Think about all the work that has been done to bring that food to our table: the farmers who grew the vegetables, the animals that gave their lives, the cooks who prepared the meal. This sense of gratitude can bring a sense of peace and fulfillment that goes beyond mere physical satiety.

Practicing Mindful Eating isn't always easy, especially in a fast-paced world where fast and convenient food is the norm. With practice and patience, we can learn to slow down, savor each bite, and nourish our body with kindness and respect. And we might find that this change not only helps us eat healthier but also improves our overall relationship with food, ourselves, and the world around us.

The journey toward Mindful Eating is a path, not a destination. Every meal is a new opportunity to practice awareness, acceptance, and respect for us.

Comfort Eating, or eating for consolation, is a common and understandable behavior. It's natural to seek relief in the small joys of life, and for many, food can offer immediate comfort. However, when food becomes too frequent a refuge, it can lead to a vicious cycle that doesn't address the underlying causes of our discomfort.

Imagine coming home after a particularly stressful day. Perhaps our first impulse is to dive into a bag of chips or a jar of ice cream. This is Comfort Eating in action. But what happens if we manage to pause that first impulse and ask ourselves, "What am I trying to heal with food?" The answer might be loneliness, frustration, nervousness, boredom, anxiety. Food cannot solve these issues, but there are many other strategies that can help.

Instead of seeking comfort in food, we can develop alternative coping methods. For instance, physical exercise can be a great alternative. Not only does it help release stress, but it also releases endorphins, chemicals that make us feel good.

Additionally, we might seek comfort in socialization. Calling a friend, spending time with family, or volunteering in our community can provide a sense of belonging and well-being.

Another effective method can be Meditation or the practice of **Mindfulness**. These techniques can help calm the mind, reduce stress, and help us recognize and address negative emotions rather than suppressing them.

It's important to remember that there's nothing wrong with finding pleasure in food. The problem arises when food becomes the only source of comfort. Ultimately, the path to a healthy relationship with food is about balance: eating to nourish our body, but also to enjoy the pleasures of the table, without it becoming a means to avoid emotional difficulties.

Comfort Eating is not an enemy to be defeated, but a signal to be listened to. It indicates that there is an unsatisfied emotional need that is asking for our attention. Let's listen to that need and try to meet it in a healthy and constructive way. This is the real secret to overcoming Comfort Eating and creating a balanced relationship with food.

The relationship between diet, self-image, and self-esteem is delicate and complex. How we perceive ourselves is influenced by countless factors, including our physical health, societal expectations, and our personal behaviors, including those related to diet.

Imagine standing in front of a mirror. What do you see? Most likely, what you'll see reflects not only your physical appearance but also how you feel about your body. If you view yourself positively, with acceptance and respect, then food will have a balanced place in your life. Conversely, if you perceive yourself negatively, food can become a battleground, a way to reward, punish, or control yourself.

Moreover, it's important to remember that our self-esteem shouldn't depend on the scale. Every person is a unique and valuable individual, regardless of weight or body shape. Restrictive diets or unrealistic beauty standards can make us feel inadequate, but these are not valid measures of our worth.

Instead of striving for an unattainable ideal, we can work to create a healthier and more positive relationship with food and ourselves. This starts with acceptance: recognizing and respecting our body for what it is and what it can do.

After acceptance, we can work to nourish our body with healthy food and physical activity, not as punishment, but as an act of love towards ourselves. Eating well and moving regularly can boost our energy, improve our mood, and help us feel more comfortable in our body.

Finally, we can adopt an attitude of gratitude. Instead of focusing on what we dislike about our body, we can choose to be grateful for what our body allows us to do: walk, run, dance, laugh. In this sense, food is a gift that enables us to fully live these experiences.

Self-image and self-esteem can be influenced by diet, but ultimately, the key to a healthy relationship with food and us lies in respect, acceptance, and gratitude. This journey isn't easy or quick, but it's worth it. After all, self-respect and self-love are the most important ingredients for a healthy and happy life.

Food and emotions have been intertwined since time immemorial. It can be comforting to reach for that cup of hot chocolate after a stressful day or celebrate a happy occasion with a special cake. It's important not to underestimate that, when food becomes our primary coping strategy for emotions—both positive and negative—it can lead to an unhealthy relationship with eating.

The art of separating emotions from food is a process that requires awareness, perseverance, and above all, a loving sense of self-compassion. It starts with recognition: understanding when the impulse to eat stems from an emotional need rather than physical hunger. This self-exploration can reveal that eating habits are tied to emotional states such as sadness, boredom, or euphoria.

Once the invisible thread connecting emotions to eating is identified, it's time to weave new strategies for tackling emotional challenges. This doesn't mean ignoring or suppressing emotions but rather learning to manage them in healthier ways.

For instance, when faced with stress, alternatives could be practicing meditation exercises, listening to your favorite music, or diving into an engaging book. If sadness overtakes you, it might be helpful to confide in a friend, write your emotions in a journal, or dedicate time to a cherished hobby. In moments of joy, you might express your happiness through dance, share the good news with your loved ones, or immerse yourself in an activity you're passionate about.

Remember, it's normal and human to experience a wide range of emotions. The goal isn't to eliminate these emotions but rather to develop a healthier and more balanced relationship with them.

Above all, be kind to yourself! Separating emotions from eating isn't easy, and there will inevitably be moments of backsliding. Instead of judging yourself harshly, remember that you're learning and that every step forward, no matter how small, is a success.

On the journey towards a more balanced relationship with food, you discover that eating isn't just a way to nourish the body, but also a way to celebrate life, enjoy pleasure, and connect with others. Moreover, it's crucial to remember that there are many other ways to respond to our emotions, ways that nourish us on all levels—physical, emotional, and spiritual—without overly depending on food.

Quote: *"Caring for myself is an act of survival." - Audre Lorde.*

CHAPTER 7

"21 Days of Wellness: Your Exciting Nutritional Plan to Transform Your Health"

We're about to embark on a 21-day journey that will transform your approach to food, not just as nourishment, but also as a source of energy, health, and wellness. This experience will be more than just a diet—it will be an odyssey of flavor, balance, and renewed food awareness.

This path, which we call "21 Days of Wellness," is a program aimed at nourishing both the body and the soul. It won't be a strict diet; instead, it's a fun and educational way to discover and experiment with new flavors. We believe every meal should be a pleasure, an opportunity to nourish the body and rejuvenate the soul.

The plan we propose offers a perfect balance of fresh fruit, vegetables, whole grains, legumes, lean proteins, and healthy fats. All ingredients that, besides being delicious, can-do wonders for your health and well-being.

Each day, you'll notice that you feel more energetic, lighter, and healthier. Your skin will start to glow, your immune system will strengthen, and your mood will improve. And most importantly, you'll begin to view food as a friend, not as an enemy.

The beauty of "21 Days of Wellness" is that it's much more than just a meal plan. It's a journey of self-discovery, a way to reconnect with your body, and to take care of yourself on a deeper level. So, are we ready? Get set to dive into this 21-day culinary adventure. It's time to nourish your health, your wellness, and your life.

Remember, although these guidelines are generally healthy, it's always a good idea to consult a healthcare professional or a nutritionist before making significant changes to your diet, especially if you have pre-existing health conditions or specific dietary needs.

Welcome to "Week 1 - Awakening the Body," your first step on this extraordinary adventure towards rejuvenated health. This week is all about one fundamental goal: awakening your body and starting the regeneration process. Here's a detailed look at what your new dietary routine could look like:

Day 1-7: Breakfast

Breakfast is the most important meal of the day, so it should be nutritious and packed with energy. To start, we suggest a bowl of homemade oatmeal, accompanied by a selection of fresh, seasonal fruits like berries, apples, or pears. Add a sprinkle of seeds, such as flax or chia seeds, which are rich in essential fatty acids and proteins. You might also add a dash of cinnamon for a touch of sweetness without the sugar.

Day 1-7: Mid-Morning Snack

A natural Greek yogurt with a handful of toasted almonds or a small apple can help keep your blood sugar stable and support your energy until lunch.

Day 1-7: Lunch

For lunch, experiment with a variety of nutrient-rich salads, incorporating a rainbow of vegetables. You can mix leafy greens like spinach or arugula with other crunchy veggies like cucumbers, bell peppers, and carrots. Add a source of protein such as chickpeas or lentils and a dressing made of extra virgin olive oil, lemon, salt, and pepper.

Day 1-7: Afternoon Snack

An afternoon snack can consist of a handful of dried fruit and nuts, or a slice of whole grain toast with a drizzle of almond butter. These foods will provide sustained energy and help you feel full until dinner.

Day 1-7: Dinner

For dinner, experiment with dishes based on whole grains like brown rice or quinoa, alongside a serving of cooked vegetables like zucchini, eggplants, or broccoli. You can try making a one-dish meal like a Buddha bowl or a buckwheat noodle dish, with sautéed veggies and a protein like tofu or tempeh.

Day 1-7: Evening Snack

If you need an evening snack, try having a fresh fruit or a small glass of unsweetened almond milk. These light foods will help ensure you don't go to bed hungry but without weighing you down.

Here is a detailed table for your first week on an anti-inflammatory diet, complete with brief recipes for each meal, portion sizes for one-person, simple cooking methods, and calorie counts:

Day	Breakfast	Mid-Morning Snack	Lunch	Afternoon Snack	Dinner	Evening Snack
1	**Oatmeal with blueberries, chia seeds, and cinnamon:** 50g oats, 100g blueberries, 10g chia seeds, a pinch of cinnamon, 250ml water or plant milk (350 kcal). Mix all ingredients and cook until creamy.	**Greek yogurt with toasted almonds:** 150g Greek yogurt, 15g toasted almonds (200 kcal). Mix and serve.	**Rainbow salad:** 30g spinach, 50g bell peppers, 50g carrots, 50g chickpeas, 1 tbsp EVOO, juice of half a lemon (300 kcal). Combine all ingredients in a bowl.	**Apple with almond butter:** 1 small apple, 10g almond butter (150 kcal). Cut the apple and spread with almond butter.	**Quinoa with sautéed vegetables and tofu:** 50g quinoa, 100g mixed vegetables (broccoli, carrots, zucchini), 50g tofu, 1 tbsp EVOO (400 kcal). Cook quinoa, sauté vegetables and tofu, and serve together.	**Almond milk:** 200ml unsweetened almond milk (30 kcal). Serve chilled.

| 2 | Oatmeal with apple and walnuts: 50g oats, 1 medium apple, 15g walnuts, 1 tbsp maple syrup, 250ml water or plant milk (370 kcal). Prepare as Day 1. | Avocado on toasted bread: 1/4 avocado, 1 slice whole-grain bread (250 kcal). Mash avocado and spread on toasted bread. | Lentil bowl: 100g cooked lentils, 50g cucumbers, 50g tomatoes, 1 tbsp EVOO, 1 tbsp balsamic vinegar (350 kcal). Mix all ingredients. | Dried fruit and nuts: 20g dried fruits, 10g nuts (150 kcal). Mix and serve. | Whole grain rice with vegetable curry: 50g whole grain rice, 150g vegetables (cauliflower, chickpeas), 100ml coconut milk, 1 tsp curry powder (450 kcal). Cook rice, make a light curry with vegetables, and serve together. | Pear: 1 medium pear (100 kcal). Serve fresh. |
| 3 | Green smoothie: 1 banana, 30g spinach, 10g flax seeds, 250ml almond milk (300 kcal). Blend all ingredients until smooth. | Cereal bar: 1 no-added-sugar bar (150 kcal). | Quinoa salad: 50g cooked quinoa, 50g cherry tomatoes, 1/4 avocado, juice of 1 lime (350 kcal). Combine all ingredients in a bowl. | Baby carrots with hummus: 100g baby carrots, 30g hummus (150 kcal). Serve carrots with hummus for dipping. | Grilled tofu with vegetables: 100g tofu, 150g mixed steamed vegetables (carrots, broccoli) (350 kcal). Grill tofu and serve with vegetables. | Kiwi: 1 kiwi (50 kcal). Serve fresh. |

4	**Oatmeal pancakes with berries:** 50g oatmeal, 100g berries, 150g Greek yogurt (400 kcal). Prepare pancakes and serve with yogurt and berries.	**Greek yogurt with honey and cinnamon:** 150g Greek yogurt, 1 teaspoon honey, a pinch of cinnamon (200 kcal). Mix and serve.	**Chicken wrap:** 100g grilled chicken, 50g lettuce, 1 tomato, 1 whole-grain wrap (350 kcal). Assemble the wrap with all ingredients.	**Almonds and dark chocolate:** 15g almonds, 10g dark chocolate (200 kcal).	**Zucchini noodles with pesto:** 200g zucchini, 30g basil and pine nut pesto (400 kcal). Prepare zucchini noodles and dress with pesto.	**Pineapple cubes:** 100g pineapple (70 kcal). Serve fresh.
5	**Spelt porridge with peaches:** 50g spelt, 1 medium peach, a pinch of nutmeg, 250ml water or plant milk (350 kcal). Cook the spelt with the peach and nutmeg.	**Berry smoothie:** 150g mixed berries, 1 teaspoon protein powder, 250ml water or plant milk (250 kcal). Blend all ingredients.	**Greek salad:** 50g lettuce, 50g cucumber, 30g olives, 50g feta, 1 tbsp EVOO (300 kcal). Combine ingredients in a bowl.	**Banana:** 1 medium banana (100 kcal).	**Baked fish with sweet potatoes:** 100g fish, 100g sweet potatoes, 100g asparagus, 1 tbsp EVOO (450 kcal). Bake the fish with the vegetables.	**Homemade banana ice cream:** 1 frozen banana blended (100 kcal). Serve immediately.
6	**Whole-grain toast with avocado:** 1 slice whole-grain bread, 1/4 avocado, 10g sunflower seeds (300 kcal). Prepare the toast with avocado and seeds.	**Mixed dried fruit:** 30g mixed dried fruit (150 kcal).	**Beetroot and orange salad:** 100g beetroots, 1 orange, 30g walnuts, 1 tbsp EVOO (350 kcal). Combine ingredients in a bowl.	**Homemade popcorn:** 30g homemade popcorn with a pinch of salt (100 kcal).	**Chicken curry with basmati rice:** 100g chicken, 50g basmati rice, 100ml coconut milk, 1 tsp curry (400 kcal). Prepare the curry with chicken and serve with rice.	**Chocolate and berry mousse:** 50g dark chocolate, 100g blueberries, 1 tsp honey, 50ml water or plant milk (250 kcal). Melt the chocolate, blend with blueberries and honey, freeze.

| 7 | Vegetable frittata: 2 eggs, 30g spinach, 50g tomatoes, 30g onions, 1 tbsp EVOO (250 kcal). Cook all vegetables and add beaten eggs. | Fresh carrot and ginger juice: 200g carrots, 10g fresh ginger (100 kcal). Extract juice from carrots and ginger. | Buddha bowl with vegetables: 50g broccoli, 50g bell peppers, 50g Brussels sprouts, 50g quinoa, 10g pumpkin seeds (400 kcal). Combine cooked ingredients in a bowl. | Rice cake with tahini: 1 whole-grain rice cake, 10g tahini (150 kcal). Spread tahini on the rice cake. | Baked salmon: 100g salmon, 50g fennel, 50g orange, 1 tbsp EVOO (350 kcal). Bake the salmon with fennel and orange. | Camomile tea: 1 cup chamomile tea (2 kcal). Prepare and serve hot. |

This plan provides a nutritional balance designed to support an anti-inflammatory diet, perfect for stimulating metabolism and reducing inflammation. Remember to adjust ingredients and portions according to your specific energy and nutritional needs.

Hydration Throughout the Day

Remember to drink water throughout the day to keep your body hydrated. Water helps flush out toxins and maintain fresh and glowing skin. Try starting your day with a glass of warm water with a bit of freshly squeezed lemon juice to boost your immune system and aid digestion.

This week's focus is not just on what you eat, but on awakening your senses to the pleasures of eating healthily and mindfully. Enjoy the journey!

During this week, we'll also focus on reducing the consumption of sugar, processed foods, and alcohol. These can inflame your body, making the healing and regeneration process more challenging. This doesn't mean you have to eliminate them entirely but try to limit their consumption as much as possible.

One of the goals this week is to introduce the "rainbow meal" practice. This concept is based on the idea that foods of different colors contain different phytonutrients that our body needs to stay healthy. So, try to include a variety of colors in every meal. For example, you could have a green vegetable like spinach, a whole grain like brown rice, a red fruit like strawberries, or an orange tuber like carrots.

Always listen to your body. Eat when you're hungry and stop when you're full. This week is the perfect time to reconnect with your feelings of hunger and satiety, which are often overlooked in the hustle and bustle of daily life. This will not only help prevent overeating but will also allow you to enjoy each meal more fully.

Know that every step you take in this direction is a step toward a healthier version of yourself. This adventure will be full of discoveries, challenges, and, hopefully, delicious meals. By the end of the week, you might already notice some changes. Perhaps you'll feel less tired, look in the mirror and see yourself more radiant, or notice that you're more in tune with your body. So, relax, enjoy the process, and let your body awaken. We hope this journey brings you joy, awareness, and a renewed appreciation for the magnificent instrument that is your body.

Welcome to "Week 2 - Consolidating Wellness," where we'll build on the foundation of well-being we established during the first week. In this phase, we'll deepen our understanding of anti-inflammatory foods and discover new ways to integrate them into our daily recipes. Here's a closer look at what your second week might look like:

Day 8-14: Breakfast

Start the day with a nutritious smoothie: a mix of fresh fruit like mango, strawberries, and blueberries, with a handful of spinach or kale to add a touch of green. Add a tablespoon of chia seeds or flax seeds for an extra dose of fiber and Omega-3 fatty acids.

Day 8-14: Mid-morning Snack

For a mid-morning snack, try a mix of nuts and seeds or a banana with a tablespoon of natural peanut butter.

Day 8-14: Lunch

For lunch, explore the world of grains: try a farro salad with cherry tomatoes, cucumbers, feta, and parsley, or a quinoa bowl with avocado, bean sprouts, and pumpkin seeds.

Day 8-14: Afternoon Snack

For an afternoon snack, experiment with homemade hummus with raw carrot sticks or peppers, or a handful of fresh cherries or blackberries.

Day 8-14: Dinner

For dinner, focus on animal proteins like salmon, tuna, or chicken. For example, try marinating salmon with a bit of raw honey, soy sauce, and ginger, or cook chicken with lemon, garlic, and rosemary. Accompany your meal with a serving of cooked vegetables like asparagus, chard, or squash.

Day 8-14: Evening Snack

If you feel like a dessert, prepare a cup of green tea or herbal tea, and accompany it with a small portion of fresh fruit or a handful of dried fruit and nuts.

Here is a detailed table for your second week of the anti-inflammatory diet, complete with brief recipes for each meal, portions for one-person, simple procedures, and calorie counts:

Day	Breakfast	Mid-Morning Snack	Lunch	Afternoon Snack	Dinner	Evening Snack
8	**Nutritious smoothie:** 100g mango, 50g strawberries, 50g blueberries, 30g spinach, 10g chia seeds, 250ml water or almond milk (300 kcal). Blend all ingredients.	**Nut and seed mix:** 20g mixed nuts, 10g sunflower seeds (150 kcal).	**Farro salad:** 50g farro, 50g cherry tomatoes, 50g cucumbers, 30g feta, 10g parsley, 1 tbsp olive oil (350 kcal). Combine and dress.	**Homemade hummus:** 30g chickpeas, 1 tbsp tahini, juice of 1/2 lemon, salt (100 kcal). Serve with 50g carrot sticks.	**Marinated salmon:** 100g salmon, 1 tbsp raw honey, 1 tbsp soy sauce, 1 tsp grated ginger, bake (400 kcal). Serve with 100g steamed asparagus.	**Green tea and fruit:** 1 cup of green tea (2 kcal), accompanied by 100g pineapple (70 kcal).
9	**Quinoa porridge:** 50g quinoa, 200ml coconut milk, 50g raspberries, 1 tsp agave syrup (350 kcal). Cook quinoa in milk, add fruit and sweetener.	**Yogurt and fresh fruit:** 150g of natural Greek yogurt, 50g of mixed berries (200 kcal). Mix the yogurt with fresh berries for a naturally sweet touch.	**Quinoa bowl:** 50g quinoa, 50g avocado, 30g soybean sprouts, 20g pumpkin seeds (300 kcal). Combine ingredients.	**Grapefruit:** 1 medium grapefruit (50 kcal).	**Lemon chicken:** 100g chicken, juice, and zest of 1 lemon, 1 clove garlic, rosemary, pan-cook (350 kcal). Serve with 100g sautéed Swiss chard.	**Herbal tea and dates:** 1 cup of herbal tea (0 kcal), accompanied by 30g dates (100 kcal).
10	**Kiwi smoothie:** 2 kiwis, 200ml soy milk, 1 tbsp flax seeds (300 kcal). Blend all ingredients.	**Homemade energy bar:** 30g oats, 10g honey, 10g almonds (200 kcal).	**Lentil salad:** 100g cooked lentils, 50g bell peppers, 1 spring onion, 1 tbsp olive oil, vinegar (300 kcal). Combine ingredients.	**Fresh cherries:** 100g cherries (70 kcal).	**Grilled tuna steak:** 100g tuna, 1 tbsp soy sauce, 1 tbsp olive oil, grill (400 kcal). Serve with 50g steamed kale.	**Almonds and dark chocolate:** 15g almonds, 10g dark chocolate (200 kcal).
11	**Overnight oats with peach:** 50g oats, 200ml almond milk, 1 medium peach, refrigerate overnight (300 kcal).	**Vegetable juice:** 200ml fresh carrot and ginger juice (100 kcal).	**Vegetable sandwich:** 2 slices whole grain bread, 50g avocado, 30g tomatoes, 20g lettuce (350 kcal). Assemble the sandwich.	**Hummus and bell peppers:** 30g hummus, 50g bell pepper strips (100 kcal).	**Grilled swordfish:** 100g swordfish, 1 tbsp olive oil, lemon, grill (350 kcal). Serve with an arugula salad (50 kcal).	**Chocolate and almond mousse:** 50g dark chocolate, 30g almonds, 50ml water or plant milk (250 kcal). Prepare as described previously.

12	Yogurt with granola and berries: 150g Greek yogurt, 30g granola, 50g berries (350 kcal). Combine ingredients.	Nuts and dried apricots: 20g nuts, 30g dried apricots (150 kcal).	Couscous bowl: 50g couscous, 50g cucumbers, 50g tomatoes, 30g feta, olive oil (350 kcal). Prepare couscous and add vegetables and feta.	Apple and peanut butter: 1 small apple, 10g peanut butter (150 kcal). Cut the apple and spread with peanut butter.	Herb chicken: 100g chicken, fresh herbs (parsley, thyme), 1 tbsp olive oil, pan-cook (400 kcal). Serve with 100g baked sweet potatoes.	Yogurt and agave syrup: 150g Greek yogurt, 1 tbsp agave syrup (200 kcal). Mix and serve.
13	Spinach and mushroom frittata: 2 eggs, 30g spinach, 50g mushrooms, 1 tbsp olive oil (300 kcal). Cook spinach and mushrooms, add beaten eggs.	Fruit and nut bar: 1 homemade bar with dates, nuts (200 kcal).	Chicken salad: 100g grilled chicken, 50g mixed salad, 30g almonds, 1 tbsp olive oil (350 kcal). Combine ingredients in a bowl.	Fresh peaches: 1 medium peach (70 kcal).	Grilled turkey steak: 100g of turkey, 1 tablespoon of extra virgin olive oil, grill (300 kcal). Serve with 50g of spinach salad.	Fruit ice cream: 100g chosen frozen fruit blended (100 kcal). Prepare and serve immediately.
14	Avocado and cocoa smoothie: 1/2 avocado, 1 tbsp cocoa powder, 250ml coconut milk, 1 tbsp agave syrup (350 kcal). Blend all ingredients.	Toasted almonds: 20g toasted almonds (150 kcal).	Turkey sandwich: 2 slices whole grain bread, 100g sliced turkey, lettuce, tomato, mustard (350 kcal). Assemble the sandwich.	Carrots and guacamole: 100g carrot sticks, 30g guacamole (150 kcal). Serve carrots with guacamole for dipping.	Baked salmon: 100g salmon, 1 tbsp raw honey, 1 tbsp mustard, bake (400 kcal). Serve with 100g	Herbal tea and oat cookies: 1 cup of herbal tea (0 kcal), 2 oat cookies (100 kcal). Prepare the tea and serve with cookies.

Each meal is calibrated to provide optimal nutritional balance, taking into account the needs of an anti-inflammatory diet. Remember to vary ingredients and portions according to your specific energy and nutritional needs.

Hydration Throughout the Day

Continue to pay attention to your hydration throughout the day. Try to vary by drinking water, green tea, herbal teas, or water infused with fresh fruit for a touch of flavor.

Reflecting on the second week encourages us to spend a bit more time on meal preparation, experimenting with new recipes, and savoring each bite. This week is also an opportunity to reconsider our relationship with sweets. Replace refined sugar with natural sweeteners like raw honey, stevia, or maple syrup.

Understand that every small change is a step towards your well-being. Nourishing your body with healthy foods is an act of self-care. Therefore, during this week, try to abandon the rush and enjoy every moment you dedicate to your nourishment. Even if challenges may arise, know that you are doing important and beneficial work for yourself.

This second week should be a time of discovery, experimentation, and appreciation. Remember to pay attention to your body's responses to these new foods and habits and make any necessary adjustments to ensure that what you're doing makes you feel good. Ultimately, the goal is not just to be healthier but also to enjoy the process of getting there.

Welcome to "Week 3 - Strengthening the Change," where we aim to cement the dietary habits cultivated and integrated into our daily routine over the past two weeks. Focus is key here:

Day 15-21: Breakfast

Experiment with a bowl of oat porridge cooked with almond or oat milk, enriched with a handful of fresh berries, chia seeds, or nuts. Alternatively, try whole-grain toast with avocado and sesame seeds.

Day 15-21: Mid-Morning Snack

Snacks are an opportunity to add more vegetables to your diet. Choose bell peppers, cucumbers, or carrots with Greek yogurt dip. For a sweet option, fresh or dried figs are great.

Day 15-21: Lunch

Introduce a different type of legume into your lunch each day. Try a lentil salad with cherry tomatoes, cucumbers, and a drizzle of olive oil, or a vegetarian chili with black beans, corn, and bell peppers.

Day 15-21: Afternoon Snack

Greek yogurt with a handful of berries and a drizzle of raw honey can be a delightful afternoon snack. For a variant, opt for a small handful of almonds and dried apricots.

Day 15-21: Dinner

For dinner, incorporate lean proteins like turkey or tofu, paired with a variety of vegetables. For example, try roasted turkey with sweet potatoes and Brussels sprouts, or stir-fried tofu with bell peppers, carrots, and broccoli.

Day 15-21: Evening Snack

Choose something light for an evening snack, like a small portion of fresh fruit. For something more substantial, an herbal tea with a teaspoon of raw honey and a whole-grain biscuit can be a good option.

This table, marking the final week of our three-week meal plan, promotes a balanced and anti-inflammatory diet, diverse and complete. It is suitable for consolidating the healthy eating habits developed in previous weeks, effectively concluding our 21-day dietary plan.

Day	Breakfast	Mid-Morning Snack	Lunch	Afternoon Snack	Dinner	Evening Snack
15	Whole grain oatmeal with almond milk: 50g oats, 250ml almond milk, 50g figs, 10g flax seeds (350 kcal). Cook oats with milk and top with figs and flax seeds.	Cucumber sticks with Greek yogurt dip: 100g cucumber, 30g Greek yogurt with herbs (100 kcal).	Lentil salad with artichokes: 100g lentils, 50g cherry tomatoes, 30g artichoke hearts, olive oil (300 kcal). Mix all ingredients with a drizzle of oil.	Greek yogurt with mango: 150g Greek yogurt, 50g mango (200 kcal).	Roasted turkey with vegetables: 100g turkey, 100g sweet potatoes, 50g Brussels sprouts, olive oil (450 kcal). Roast the turkey and vegetables.	Herbal tea with whole grain biscuit: 1 cup herbal tea, 1 whole grain biscuit (100 kcal).

16	Buckwheat pancakes: 50g buckwheat flour, 100ml oat milk, 1 egg (300 kcal). Make pancakes and serve with maple syrup.	Fresh figs: 2 fresh figs (90 kcal).	Vegetarian chili: 50g black beans, 50g corn, 100g bell peppers, tomatoes, onions (350 kcal). Cook all ingredients together.	Dried apricots and almonds: 30g dried apricots, 15g almonds (150 kcal).	Tofu stir-fry: 100g tofu, 50g bell peppers, 50g carrots, 50g broccoli, soy sauce (400 kcal). Stir-fry the tofu and vegetables with a bit of soy sauce.	Fresh apple: 1 medium apple (80 kcal).
17	Homemade cereal bar: 30g oats, 15g pumpkin seeds, 10g honey, 10g almonds (250 kcal). Prepare and bake the bars.	Carrots with avocado dip: 100g carrots, 30g mashed avocado seasoned with lime juice and a pinch of salt (150 kcal).	Cannellini bean salad: 100g cannellini beans, 50g arugula, 30g cherry tomatoes, olive oil (300 kcal). Combine ingredients with a drizzle of oil.	Banana and strawberry smoothie: 1 banana, 50g strawberries, 200ml soy milk (250 kcal). Blend all ingredients.	Baked salmon with asparagus: 100g salmon, chives, lemon, olive oil (400 kcal). Serve the salmon baked with chives and lemon, accompanied by 100g of steamed asparagus.	Greek yogurt with raspberries: 150g Greek yogurt, 50g raspberries (150 kcal).
18	Apple and cinnamon smoothie: 1 apple, 200ml almond milk, cinnamon (250 kcal). Blend all ingredients.	Greek yogurt with granola: 150g Greek yogurt, 30g granola (200 kcal).	Quinoa salad with eggplant: 50g cooked quinoa, 50g roasted eggplant, 50g tomatoes, lime juice, fresh basil (350 kcal). Mix fresh ingredients with cooked quinoa.	Almonds and blueberries: 15g almonds, 30g blueberries (150 kcal).	Grilled swordfish: 100g swordfish, lemon, parsley, olive oil (400 kcal). Grill the fish with lemon and parsley.	Cup of mallow tea: 1 cup (2 kcal). Serve hot.
19	Apple and cinnamon smoothie: 1 apple, 200ml almond milk, cinnamon (250 kcal). Blend all ingredients.	Greek yogurt with granola: 150g Greek yogurt, 30g granola (200 kcal).	Vegetarian sandwich: 2 slices of whole grain bread, 50g of mashed avocado, slices of bell peppers, arugula, and shredded	Almonds and blueberries: 15g almonds, 30g blueberries (150 kcal).	Grilled swordfish: 100g swordfish, lemon, parsley, olive oil (400 kcal). Grill the fish with lemon and parsley.	Cup of peppermint tea: 1 cup (2 kcal). Serve hot.

			carrots (300 kcal). Assemble the sandwich with these fresh vegetables for a crunchy and flavorful meal.			
20	**Turmeric vegetable omelette:** 2 eggs, 50g zucchini, 30g asparagus, 1 tsp turmeric, 1 tbsp olive oil (300 kcal). Prepare the omelette with sautéed zucchini and asparagus, seasoned with turmeric.	**Orange segments:** 1 medium orange (80 kcal).	**Buddha bowl with tofu:** 50g tofu, 50g broccoli, 50g carrots, 50g cauliflower, 50g whole rice, soy sauce (350 kcal). Assemble the Buddha bowl with all ingredients.	**Fruit sorbet:** 100g frozen blended fruit (100 kcal).	**Baked turkey with vegetables:** 100g turkey, 100g zucchini, 50g carrots, thyme, olive oil (450 kcal). Bake the turkey with vegetables.	**Mango and ginger mousse:** 1 ripe mango, 1 tsp freshly grated ginger, 1 tsp honey, 200ml coconut milk (250 kcal). Blend all ingredients until smooth and serve chilled.
21	**Toast with ricotta and tomatoes:** 2 slices of whole grain bread, 50g ricotta, 50g sliced tomatoes, basil (300 kcal). Prepare the toast with ricotta, tomatoes, and basil.	**Mixed nuts and seeds:** 20g walnuts, 10g sunflower seeds (150 kcal).	**Chickpea and spinach salad:** 100g chickpeas, 50g spinach, 30g sun-dried tomatoes, olive oil, balsamic vinegar (300 kcal). Combine ingredients in a bowl.	**Fresh peaches:** 1 medium peach (70 kcal).	**Baked cod with herbs:** 100g cod, fresh herbs (basil, parsley), lemon, olive oil (400 kcal). Bake the cod with herbs and lemon.	**Oat cookies:** 2 homemade oat cookies (100 kcal).

Hydration Throughout the Day

Don't forget to maintain good hydration levels throughout the day. Drink fresh water, green tea, herbal teas, and try varying with infused water with slices of fresh fruit or mint leaves for a flavor twist.

Physical Activity

Incorporate physical activity into your daily schedule. A 30-minute walk per day, swimming, cycling, or any other activity you enjoy can make a big difference in your overall well-being.

Reflection on the Third Week

During this week, continue to reflect on your food choices and lifestyle modifications. Remember, the goal is to build a long-term health and wellness journey.

Keep cultivating a positive relationship with food, seeing it as a means to nourish your body and support your health. Make room for gratitude, appreciating the nutrients you're providing your body and the benefits you're gaining. Celebrate the progress you're making and recognize the value of every small step forward.

Don't be discouraged if you encounter obstacles or setbacks. These are normal and part of the change process. The important thing is not to get discouraged, but to learn from these experiences and use them to strengthen your resolve.

Well-being is not a destination, but a continuous journey. With commitment, determination, and a positive attitude, you can transform challenges into opportunities and keep moving toward your goal of a healthier, happier life.

To summarize, during the third week, your focus will be on reinforcing the changes you made in the previous two weeks by incorporating even more nutritious and healthy foods into your diet, staying well-hydrated, maintaining a physical exercise routine, and continuing to develop your awareness and approach to food.

Do your best to plan your meals in advance and prepare them with fresh, nutritious ingredients. Experiment with new recipes and flavors, encouraging variety in your diet. Replace processed and high-sugar foods with healthier, more nutrient-rich options. Listen to your body and adapt your meal plan according to its needs.

Keep up the great work, because you're on the right path to achieving your goal of a healthier and happier lifestyle.

Here's a list of some anti-inflammatory foods for your 21-day journey or for life. These foods will also be found in the next chapters dedicated to recipes that I hope you'll enjoy! Experiment with them as they are or change the ingredients to your liking, personal taste, and physical needs.

Fruit: Blueberries, Cherries, Pineapple, Avocado, Apples, Pear, Grapes, Oranges, Bananas, Kiwi, Raspberries, Papaya, Grapefruit, Peaches, Plums, Figs, Melons, Watermelon, Strawberries, Apricots, Pomegranate.

Vegetables: Spinach, Kale, Broccoli, Peppers, Tomatoes, Beets, Cauliflower, Carrots, Zucchini, Arugula, Asparagus, Sweet potatoes, Cucumbers, Swiss chard, Celery, Cabbage, Brussels sprouts, Peas, Lettuce, Mushrooms, Seaweed.

Fish: Salmon, Tuna, Sardines, Anchovies, Trout, Sea bass, Gilthead, Swordfish, Cod, Puffer fish, Blue fish, Mullet, Bass, Squid, Shrimp.

White Meats: Chicken, Turkey, Rabbit, Guinea fowl, Pheasant, Hen.

Allowed Sugars: Manuka honey, Raw honey, Stevia, Pure maple syrup, Coconut sugar, Yacon syrup, Molasses, Agave syrup.

Cereals and Legumes: Oats, Quinoa, Spelt, Lentils, Chickpeas, Beans, Bulgur, Amaranth, Peas, Fava beans, Borlotti beans, Buckwheat, Millet, Black beans, Cannellini beans, Red lentils, Seitan.

Rice: Basmati, Brown, Black, Whole red rice, Wild rice, Venere rice, Carnaroli rice, Arborio rice.

Pasta: Spelt pasta, Whole grain rice pasta, Quinoa pasta, Kamut pasta, Whole spelt pasta, Legume pasta, Buckwheat pasta, Millet pasta, Corn pasta, Gluten-free pasta.

Cheeses: Feta, Goat cheese, Ricotta, Buffalo mozzarella, Greek yogurt, Soy cheese (tofu).

Milk Alternatives: Coconut milk, Oat milk, Almond milk, Rice milk, Soy milk, Hazelnut milk.

Oily Seeds: Flax seeds, Chia seeds, Pumpkin seeds, Almonds, Walnuts, Sunflower seeds, Sesame seeds, Hazelnuts, Poppy seeds, Brazil nuts, Pecan nuts, Cumin seeds, Fennel seeds.

Spices: Ginger, Cumin, Saffron, Turmeric, Black pepper, Cinnamon, Cloves, Nutmeg, Paprika.

Aromatic Herbs: Parsley, Basil, Oregano, Rosemary, Sage, Thyme, Mint, Dill, Coriander.

Plants: Cocoa, Green tea, Matcha, Rooibos, Ginseng, Chamomile, Mallow.

These foods will bring a breath of freshness to your diet and help maintain low levels of inflammation in your body. Enjoy your meal! And let your adventure begin Now!

RECIPES

CHAPTER 5

Quote: "Life is too short to skip breakfast." - John Gunther.

CHAPTER 8

"Tasty Dawn: Breakfasts for a Flavorful Awakening"

Step into the dimension of "Tasty Dawn," a parallel universe where waking up is not just a simple transition from the world of dreams to reality, but an opportunity to celebrate with an explosion of flavors and nutrients. Every dawn here brings with it the prospect of a new day, a potential that deserves to be greeted with a meal that nourishes both body and soul.

In this world, waking up is not a duty, but a vibrant anticipation, a thrill of anticipation for the culinary feast that awaits. And as you live this moment, keep in mind that we're talking not just about flavors and aromas. It's an adventure through different nuances, the interplay between hot and cold, sweet, and salty, creamy, and crunchy.

We will experience the magic of smoothies, a true river of vitality trapped in a simple glass, a fusion of anti-inflammatory ingredients working in symbiosis to revitalize your body. And then, why not dive into a sea of delicious porridge, or discover new worlds with pancakes. We will listen to the crunchy melody of bruschettas and toasts, both sweet and salty, and dance with omelets and frittatas. Each one a chapter of a timeless recipe book, just waiting to be written.

In this chapter of "Tasty Dawn," the focus is not just on a moment of the day. We are talking about a philosophy of life that starts with the first meal of the day. A way of approaching nutrition that encourages reflection on what we eat and how our choices can energize the day. So, let's prepare to contemplate the dawn with a renewed sense of wonder and enjoyment - because a flavorful awakening is the prelude to an extraordinary day.

"Extraordinary Smoothies"

"Emerald Embrace Smoothie"

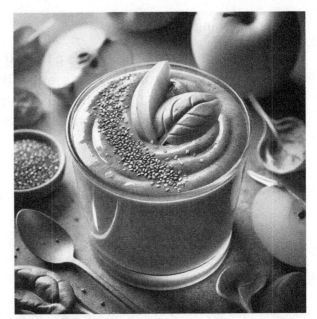

Ingredients for 1 person:

1 green apple

1 small piece of fresh ginger (about 1 cm)

1 teaspoon of turmeric powder

A handful of fresh spinach

1 glass of unsweetened almond milk

1 tablespoon of chia seeds

Juice of half a lemon

Procedure: Thoroughly wash the apple and fresh spinach. There's no need to peel the apple; its skin contains valuable antioxidants. Cut the apple into small pieces and put it in the blender.

Continue with the ginger. Peel it and slice it thinly, then add it to the blender. Now, add the turmeric powder, a true concentrate of well-being.

It's time for the spinach. These green leaves are an invaluable source of nutrients and have an anti-inflammatory action. Add them to the blender.

Perfect, now pour in the almond milk. This plant-based milk is a great alternative to cow's milk, naturally sweet, and rich in vitamin E, a powerful antioxidant.

Add the chia seeds for an extra dose of fiber, protein, and Omega-3 fatty acids, which have an important anti-inflammatory action.

Finish with the juice of half a lemon, which not only adds a touch of freshness but also helps with the absorption of turmeric.

Blend everything until smooth.

Benefits: The "Emerald Embrace" is a true elixir of life: rich in antioxidants from the apple, ginger, and turmeric, it has anti-inflammatory properties thanks to the spinach and chia seeds. The almond milk provides vitamin E, while the lemon enhances the absorption of turmeric. A smoothie that invigorates, nourishes, and fights inflammation.

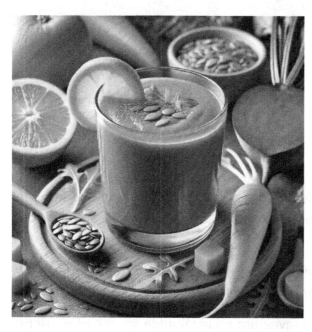

"Wake Up the Senses Smoothie"

Ingredients for 1 person:

1 small red beet

1 carrot

1 orange

1 teaspoon of flaxseeds

1 teaspoon of pumpkin seeds

1 glass of coconut water

Procedure: Begin by thoroughly washing the beet and carrot. Cut them into pieces and put them in the blender.

Continue with the orange. Use a sharp knife to peel it, then cut it into pieces and add it to the blender.

Add the flaxseeds and pumpkin seeds. These seeds are rich in Omega-3 fatty acids and have an important anti-inflammatory action. Additionally, pumpkin seeds are an excellent source of magnesium, which is essential for heart health and mood.

Now, pour in the coconut water. This natural drink, with its sweet and refreshing flavor, is rich in electrolytes that help maintain the body's hydration, very important for overall well-being.

Blend everything until smooth and creamy. If you wish, you can add some ice to make it even more refreshing.

Benefits: "Wake Up the Senses" is a symphony of nutrients and flavor: the beet and carrot bring fiber and vitamins, while the orange provides a powerful dose of vitamin C. The flaxseeds and pumpkin seeds are rich in anti-inflammatory Omega-3s and magnesium. Finally, the coconut water adds hydration and essential minerals. A smoothie that awakens the senses and rejuvenates the body.

"Tropical Sun Smoothie"

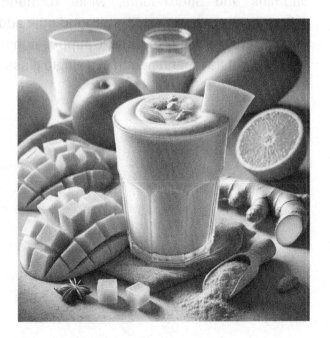

Ingredients for 1 person:

1 ripe mango

1 orange

1 teaspoon of turmeric powder

1 teaspoon of grated fresh ginger

200 ml of almond milk

A pinch of black pepper (helps with the absorption of turmeric)

Procedure: First, peel the mango and orange. For the mango, remember to remove the pit. For the orange, try to remove the white part as well, which could make the smoothie slightly bitter.

Cut the fruits into pieces and put them in the blender.

Add the turmeric and grated ginger. Fresh ginger, besides adding a spicy touch to the smoothie, is a powerful natural anti-inflammatory.

Pour the almond milk into the blender. If you want a thicker smoothie, reduce the amount of milk.

Add a pinch of black pepper. This step might seem unusual, but black pepper helps our body absorb turmeric, making this smoothie even healthier.

Blend everything until smooth and creamy. If necessary, add some water or more almond milk to reach the desired consistency.

Pour the smoothie into a glass and enjoy your "Tropical Sun"!

Benefits: "Tropical Sun" is a cocktail of well-being: mango and orange are rich in vitamins and antioxidants, while turmeric and ginger offer powerful anti-inflammatory properties. The almond milk adds creaminess and nourishes with its plant proteins, while the black pepper enhances the absorption of turmeric. An explosion of flavor and health in a single glass.

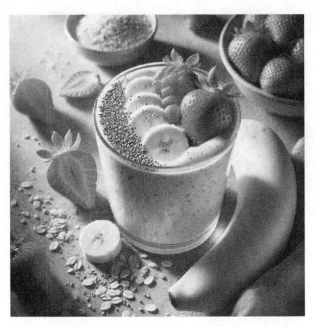

"Morning Harmony Smoothie"

Ingredients for 1 person:

1 ripe banana

1 cup of fresh strawberries

1 tablespoon of chia seeds

200 ml of oat milk

1 teaspoon of honey (optional)

Procedure: Peel the banana and slice it. Wash the strawberries well, remove the stems, and cut them in half. Put the fruits in the blender.

Add the chia seeds to the mix. These small seeds are a concentrate of nutrients and have anti-inflammatory properties.

Pour the oat milk into the blender. This type of milk is a great plant-based alternative, rich in fiber and with a low glycemic index.

Add a teaspoon of honey for a touch of natural sweetness. This step is optional and can be omitted if you prefer a less sweet taste or if you are trying to reduce sugar in your diet.

Blend everything until you get a smooth and creamy smoothie. If you want a more liquid smoothie, add some water or more oat milk. Pour the smoothie into a glass and serve.

Benefits: "Morning Harmony" is a nutritious and balanced recipe: the banana provides energy and potassium, strawberries are an excellent source of vitamin C and antioxidants, chia seeds offer fiber, protein, and Omega-3 fatty acids, while oat milk contributes with plant proteins and a low glycemic index. Together, these ingredients create a delicious and healthy meal.

"Dive into Green Smoothie"

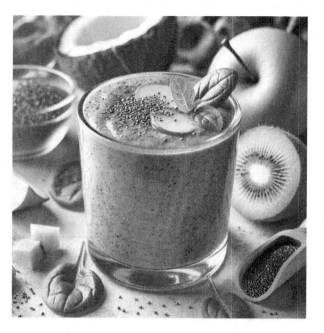

Ingredients for 1 person:

1 green apple, cut into pieces and cored

1/2 cucumber, cut into pieces

2 kiwis, peeled and cut into pieces

A handful of fresh spinach

A small piece of fresh ginger, peeled and grated

1 teaspoon of chia seeds

1 cup of coconut water (or plain filtered water, if you prefer)

Procedure: First, prepare the fruit and vegetables. Cut the green apple, cucumber, and kiwis into pieces. Remember to remove the core from the apple. Grate the fresh ginger.

Place the green apple, cucumber, kiwis, fresh spinach, grated ginger, chia seeds, and coconut water in a blender.

Blend all ingredients together until you get a smooth and homogeneous mixture. If you want a thinner smoothie, you can add a little more water.

Pour the smoothie into a large glass and enjoy it immediately, to make the most of the nutritional properties of the ingredients.

Benefits: The result is a detoxifying green smoothie, fresh and nutritious, perfect to start the day. Coconut water (or filtered water) provides hydration, while the fruit and vegetables provide vitamins, minerals, and fiber. Chia seeds add an extra touch of protein and fiber, and ginger adds a spicy note that helps to stimulate metabolism. A real dive into green for an energetic and nutritious wake-up. Enjoy your breakfast!

"Exotic Dawn Smoothie"

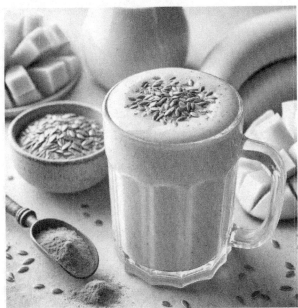

Ingredients for 1 person:

1 ripe banana, peeled and chopped

1 mango, peeled and chopped

2 tablespoons of flax seeds

1 cup of oat milk

1 teaspoon of turmeric powder

A pinch of black pepper (optional, but recommended to enhance the absorption of turmeric)

Procedure: Start by preparing the fruit: peel and chop the banana and mango.

In a blender, add the banana, mango, flax seeds, turmeric, and oat milk.

Blend everything together until you achieve a smooth and creamy consistency. If you prefer a more liquid smoothie, you can add a little more oat milk.

Lastly, add a pinch of black pepper. This step is optional, but the pepper helps the body absorb the turmeric, thus enhancing its anti-inflammatory effects.

Pour the smoothie into a glass and enjoy it immediately to benefit from the nutritional properties of the ingredients.

Benefits: This creamy smoothie, rich in nutrients and natural anti-inflammatories, is perfect for an energy-filled start to the day. The sweet, tropical taste of banana and mango is balanced by the slight spiciness of turmeric, while the oat milk gives it a smooth, creamy consistency. The flax seeds add fiber and omega-3, making this smoothie a complete and nutritious meal. Good morning!

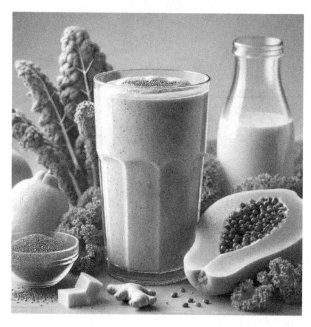

"Morning Sprint Smoothie"

Ingredients for 1 person:

1 medium papaya, peeled and seeded

A bunch of kale (curly), washed and stemless

1 lemon, juiced

A piece of fresh ginger, peeled (about 1 cm)

250 ml of unsweetened almond milk

1 tablespoon of chia seeds

Procedure: Begin by preparing all the ingredients. Clean the papaya well, remove the seeds, and cut it into pieces. Also prepare the kale by removing the tougher stems.

Put the papaya, kale, lemon juice, ginger, and almond milk in a blender. Blend until smooth.

Add the chia seeds and blend again for a couple of seconds, just enough to mix the seeds well into the smoothie.

Pour the smoothie into a large glass and enjoy it immediately to make the most of the nutritional benefits of this energy drink.

Benefits: This smoothie is not only an explosion of tropical flavors but also a true concentrate of health benefits. Papaya is rich in vitamins A and C, kale is a superfood with a high content of vitamin K and iron, ginger is known for its anti-inflammatory properties, almond milk provides plant proteins, and chia seeds are a source of fiber and omega-3. A true wellness cocktail in a glass.

"Blue Explosion Smoothie"

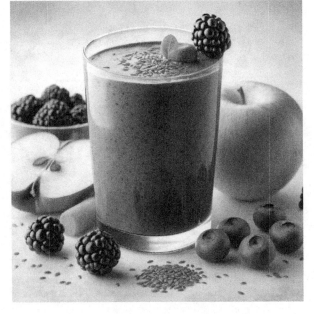

Ingredients for 1 person:

1 cup of blackberries, fresh or frozen

1 apple, cut into pieces

1 carrot, cut into pieces

250 ml of unsweetened coconut milk

1 tablespoon of flaxseeds

1 teaspoon of honey (optional)

Procedure: Prepare all the ingredients. If you're using frozen blackberries, there's no need to thaw them beforehand. Wash and cut the apple and carrot into pieces.

Place the blackberries, apple, carrot, coconut milk, and flaxseeds in a blender. Blend until you achieve a smooth and creamy consistency.

Taste and decide if you want to add a bit of sweetness with a teaspoon of honey. If so, blend again for a couple of seconds to incorporate the honey well.

Pour the smoothie into a glass and enjoy immediately. You can also put the smoothie in the fridge for a while if you prefer a colder drink.

Benefits: This "Blue Explosion" smoothie is a true concentrate of antioxidants thanks to the blackberries, while the coconut milk provides an exotic touch and a dose of good fats. The apple and carrot add natural sweetness and additional nutrients, and the flaxseeds provide fiber and omega-3. A delicious and nutritious way to start the day!

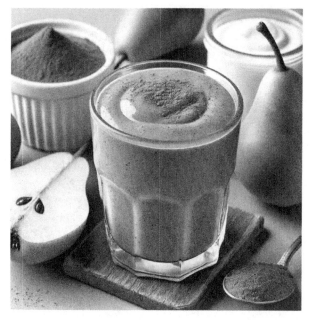

"A Glass of Vitality Smoothie"

Ingredients for 1 person:

1 ripe pear, preferably organic

2 level tablespoons of unsweetened cocoa powder

200 grams of unsweetened Greek yogurt

Procedure: Wash the pear, remove the core, and cut it into pieces, leaving the skin on as it is rich in fiber.

In a blender, combine the chopped pear, cocoa powder, and Greek yogurt.

Blend until you achieve a smooth and creamy mixture. If necessary, you can add a little water to reach the desired consistency.

Serve immediately to fully enjoy the freshness of the ingredients.

Benefits: This recipe is a concentrate of health: the pear provides fiber and vitamins, the bitter cocoa is rich in antioxidants, and the Greek yogurt contributes proteins and probiotics. Together, they create a creamy and delicious beverage, capable of energizing and, thanks to the anti-inflammatory properties of the ingredients, contributing to the well-being of the organism. A glass of this smoothie represents a start of the day full of vitality or a rejuvenating snack during the day.

"Comfortable Awakening Porridge"

"Energizing Wake-Up Porridge"

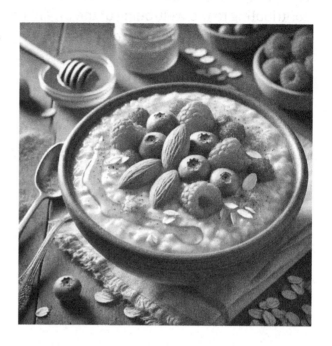

Ingredients for 2 people:

1 cup of oat flakes

2 cups of almond milk

1 teaspoon of turmeric powder

A pinch of black pepper

1 tablespoon of honey

A handful of toasted almonds

A handful of red fruits (such as raspberries, blueberries, or strawberries)

Procedure: Start by mixing the oat flakes and almond milk in a saucepan. Oats are an extraordinary food offering fiber, protein, and a range of vitamins and minerals, while almond milk is a great alternative to traditional milk for those following a plant-based diet.

Bring the mixture to a boil, then reduce the heat and simmer for 10-15 minutes, until the oats have softened, and the milk has been absorbed.

Add turmeric powder and a pinch of black pepper. Turmeric is a powerful anti-inflammatory, and the addition of black pepper helps the body absorb it better.

Stir well, then turn off the heat and let it cool for a few minutes.

Distribute the oats into two bowls, then season with a tablespoon of honey for natural sweetness.

Finally, add a handful of toasted almonds for some crunchiness and a handful of red fruits for a burst of flavor and antioxidants.

Serve hot and enjoy this delicious breakfast that offers a perfect balance of nutrients to start the day with energy!

Benefits: The "Energizing Wake-Up" combines oats, rich in fiber for digestive health, and turmeric, a potent anti-inflammatory. The almonds add a dose of protein and healthy fats, while the red fruits offer vital antioxidants. The result is an energizing and healthful breakfast.

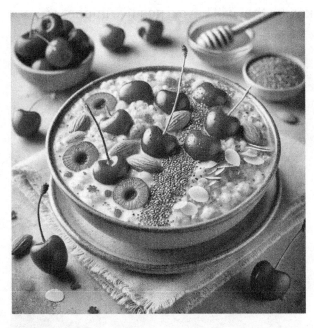

"Cherry Blossom Porridge"

Ingredients for 1 person:

1 cup of puffed spelt

1/2 cup of almond milk

2 tablespoons of raw honey

1 cup of fresh cherries, pitted and halved

1 tablespoon of chia seeds

1 tablespoon of almond flakes

1 teaspoon of vanilla extract

Procedure: Pour the almond milk into a large bowl, add the honey and vanilla extract, and stir until the honey has completely dissolved.

Add the puffed spelt to the bowl, mixing well to ensure it soaks up the milk mixture.

Add the halved fresh cherries, chia seeds, and almond flakes. Mix well.

Let the mixture rest for about 15 minutes, so the puffed spelt can soften.

Serve your "Cherry Blossom" bowl with an extra sprinkle of chia seeds or almond flakes, if desired.

Benefits: This delicious dish is packed with health and vitality. Cherries are rich in antioxidants and vitamin C, useful for fighting inflammation and strengthening the immune system. The puffed spelt provides fibers that aid digestion and give a prolonged sense of fullness. Finally, almond milk, chia seeds, and almonds provide essential fatty acids, proteins, and calcium, helping to keep muscles strong and bones firm. A nutritious and tasty awakening that will have a positive impact on your day.

"Apricot Sweet Awakening Porridge"

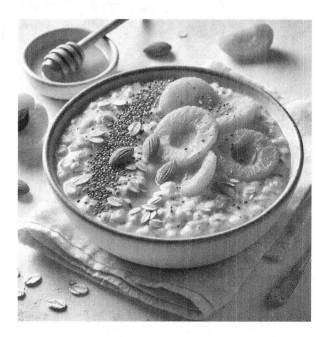

Ingredients for 1 person:

Whole oat flakes, 40-50 grams

Almond milk, 200 ml

Honey, 1 tablespoon

Dried apricots, 4-5 pieces

Chia seeds, 1 tablespoon

Procedure: Start with a serving of whole oat flakes, about 40-50 grams, in a large bowl. Oat flakes are an ideal food to start the day, as they are rich in fiber, proteins, and complex carbohydrates that release energy gradually.

Pour 200 ml of almond milk over the oat flakes. Almond milk, in addition to being a plant-based source of calcium, has a lower caloric content compared to cow's milk, and is rich in vitamin E, a powerful antioxidant.

Add a tablespoon of honey to sweeten. Honey is a natural sweetener, rich in antioxidants, and has antibacterial and anti-inflammatory properties.

Add 4-5 chopped dried apricots. Dried apricots are an excellent source of vitamins A and C and contain antioxidants and fibers.

Finish with a sprinkle of chia seeds, which provide fiber, proteins, and omega-3 fatty acids.

Mix everything together and let the bowl rest in the refrigerator for at least an hour, or overnight. The following morning, you will find a filling and nutritious meal ready to be enjoyed.

Benefits: The "Apricot Sweet Awakening" is a balanced, nutritious, and flavorful breakfast. The energy from the oats, the anti-inflammatory effect of honey, the vitamins from the apricots, and the benefits of almonds and chia seeds combine to offer you a breakfast that can contribute to healthy digestion, strengthen the immune system, and provide energy for the entire day. Enjoy your meal!

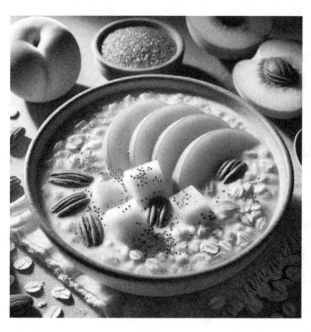

"Sunbeam Porridge"

Ingredients for 2 people:

1 cup of rolled oats

2 cups of coconut milk

1 ripe peach

2 slices of fresh pineapple

2 teaspoons of honey or maple syrup

1 tablespoon of chia seeds

A handful of pecan nuts or almond flakes

Procedure: In a saucepan, add the rolled oats and coconut milk. Bring to a boil then reduce the heat, simmering until the oats have absorbed most of the liquid and softened, about 10-15 minutes.

Meanwhile, halve the peach, remove the stone, and slice thinly. Cut the pineapple into equally sized pieces.

Once the oats are cooked, stir in the honey or maple syrup well.

Serve the warm oats in bowls, garnished with peach slices, pineapple pieces, chia seeds, and pecan nuts or almond flakes.

If desired, you can add a little extra coconut milk over each serving to make it even creamier.

Benefits: The "Sunbeam Porridge" recipe is a burst of nutrients: oats provide fiber and protein, promoting satiety and heart health. Coconut milk adds a tropical touch and contains medium-chain fatty acids, useful for energy. Peach and pineapple offer vitamins, minerals, and antioxidants, essential for the immune system. Chia seeds are rich in fiber, protein, and Omega-3, while pecan nuts and almonds add proteins and healthy fats.

"Relaxed Home Atmosphere Pancakes"

"Tropical Morning Pancakes"

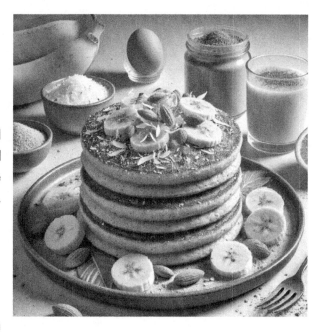

For this recipe, you should yield about 3 to 4 medium-sized pancakes, depending on the amount of batter used for each one.

1 cup of almond flour

2 eggs

1 ripe banana

1 teaspoon of unsweetened cocoa powder

2 tablespoons of dehydrated coconut flakes

1 teaspoon of baking powder

A pinch of salt

Almond milk to achieve the desired consistency

Procedure: Mash the banana with a fork until it becomes pureed. In a bowl, mix the almond flour with the cocoa, baking powder, and salt. In another bowl, beat the eggs, add the mashed banana, and mix.

Combine the egg and banana mixture with the dry ingredients, mixing until you obtain a uniform batter. Gradually add almond milk until you reach the desired consistency for your pancakes.

Heat a non-stick pan and pour a ladle of pancake batter onto it. Cook each pancake for 2-3 minutes per side, or until they turn golden. Repeat until the batter is used up. Decorate the pancakes with coconut flakes.

Benefits: "Tropical Morning" is a delicious and nutritious breakfast. The almond flour provides proteins and healthy fats, while the banana offers fiber and potassium. The cocoa adds a touch of flavor without added sugars, and the coconut flakes provide an additional layer of texture and flavor. A dish that envelops the palate with a tropical taste and ensures a balanced and sustainable energy intake for the entire morning.

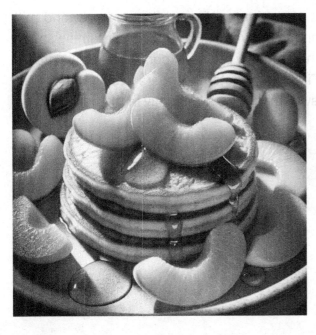

"Morning Light Pancakes"

For this recipe, you should get about 3/4 medium-sized pancakes, depending on the amount of batter used for each.

1 cup of almond flour

1/2 cup of almond milk

2 large eggs

1 teaspoon of baking powder

1 teaspoon of vanilla extract

A pinch of salt

2 apricots or 1 large pear

Maple syrup, for garnish

Procedure: In a bowl, mix the almond flour, baking powder, and salt.

In another bowl, whisk together the eggs, almond milk, and vanilla extract.

Gradually add the dry ingredients to the wet ones, mixing until you get a smooth and homogeneous batter. Cut the apricots or pear into thin slices.

Preheat a non-stick skillet over medium heat and add some coconut oil or vegetable butter.

Pour a ladle of batter into the skillet for each pancake. Add a few slices of fruit on top of the batter. Cook until the surface begins to bubble; then flip it and cook for another minute or two. Serve the pancakes warm with maple syrup and the remaining fresh fruit.

Benefits: An incredible breakfast full of nutrients. Almond flour and almond milk provide a generous dose of proteins and healthy fats, useful for maintaining satiety throughout the day. Eggs, a source of high-quality proteins, contribute to the growth and maintenance of muscle mass. Finally, apricots and pears provide fibers and essential vitamins, offering a natural sweetness to start the day in the best way.

"Sweet Awakening Pancakes"

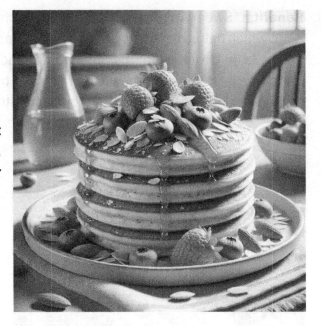

For this recipe, you should get about 3/4 medium-sized pancakes, depending on the amount of batter used for each.

1 cup of oat flour

2 eggs

1/2 cup of Greek yogurt

1 teaspoon of ground cinnamon

2 tablespoons of honey

1/2 cup of chopped almonds

Olive oil for cooking

Fresh fruit of your choice

Procedure: In a large bowl, combine the oat flour, eggs, Greek yogurt, and cinnamon. Mix well until you get a homogeneous batter. Add the honey to the batter and mix again.

Heat a non-stick skillet over medium heat and add a drizzle of olive oil.

Use a ladle to pour the batter into the skillet, creating pancakes about 10 cm in diameter.

Cook the pancakes for 2-3 minutes per side, or until golden brown.

Once cooked, transfer the pancakes to a plate and sprinkle them with the chopped almonds.

Serve the pancakes warm, accompanied by honey or fresh fruit of your choice.

Benefits: "Sweet Awakening" is a nutrient-rich and fiber-rich recipe thanks to the oat flour, which helps regulate digestion and keeps you fuller for longer. The eggs provide high-quality proteins for tissue maintenance. Greek yogurt, rich in probiotics, promotes intestinal health, while cinnamon has antioxidant and anti-inflammatory properties. Finally, the almonds provide healthy fats for the heart.

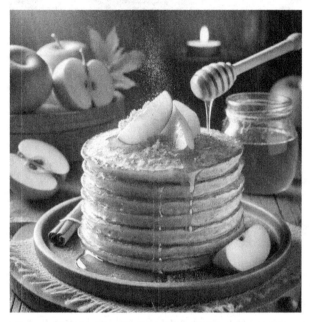

"Autumn Pancakes"

For this recipe, you should be able to make about 3/4 medium-sized pancakes, depending on the amount of batter you use for each.

1 cup of rice flour

1 large apple

1 egg

1 teaspoon of ground cinnamon

1 teaspoon of baking powder

1 tablespoon of coconut oil

1/2 cup of almond milk (or another plant-based drink)

Procedure: Start by grating the apple and set it aside. In a bowl, combine the rice flour, cinnamon, and baking powder. In another bowl, beat the egg with the almond milk.

Pour the wet ingredients into the dry ingredients and mix until you get a smooth batter. Add the grated apple and mix again.

Heat a non-stick skillet and lightly grease with a bit of coconut oil. Pour a ladle of batter for each pancake, cooking until bubbles form on the surface, then flip it over and cook on the other side. Serve your pancakes with a drizzle of maple syrup or honey, if desired.

Benefits: These pancakes are not only delicious but, thanks to the apples and cinnamon, can help regulate blood sugar, while the rice flour makes them light and digestible. Ideal for a tasty and healthy awakening.

"Bruschetta & Toast: Robust and Genuine Flavors for a Fragrant Morning"

"Sweet-Salty Morning Embrace Bruschetta"

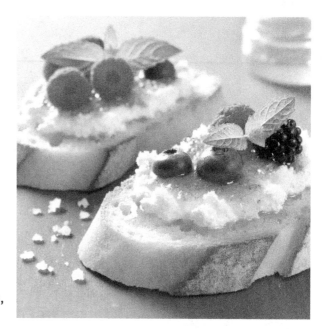

Ingredients for 2 people:

2 slices of homemade bread

100g of fresh ricotta

1 tablespoon of honey

1 cup of mixed berries (raspberries, blueberries, blackberries)

A pinch of salt

Fresh mint for garnish

Procedure: First, toast the bread slices in a toaster or in the oven at 180°C until they become golden and crispy.

Meanwhile, mix the ricotta with honey and a pinch of salt in a bowl until creamy.

Gently wash the berries and dry them.

Once the bread is ready, spread it generously with the ricotta and honey cream.

Distribute the berries over the ricotta, ensuring they are evenly distributed.

Garnish with some fresh mint leaves.

Benefits: This morning bruschetta provides a great source of proteins thanks to the ricotta, which can help keep you full longer. The berries are packed with antioxidants, beneficial for heart and brain health. Finally, honey provides natural sweetness and has antibacterial properties.

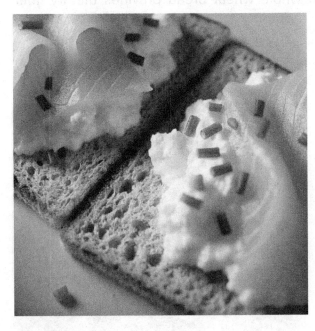

"Nutrient Ray Toast"

Ingredients for 2 people:

2 slices of whole wheat bread

4 eggs

100g smoked salmon

2 tablespoons almond milk

1 tablespoon extra-virgin olive oil

Salt and pepper

Fresh chives

Procedure: Start by toasting the slices of whole wheat bread in a toaster or in the oven at 180°C (356°F) for 5 minutes.

While the bread is toasting, crack the eggs into a bowl, add the almond milk, a pinch of salt and pepper. Whisk well until the mixture becomes homogeneous.

Heat a little olive oil in a non-stick pan over medium heat. Once hot, pour the egg and milk mixture. Let it cook for a minute without stirring, then start gently folding with a spatula, creating soft folds.

Continue cooking until the eggs are no longer liquid, but still creamy. Remove from heat.

Distribute the smoked salmon on the toasted bread slices, then top with the scrambled eggs. Garnish with some chopped chives.

Benefits: This morning toast is rich in proteins provided by the eggs and salmon, which can help maintain strong muscles and promote satiety. Salmon is also a great source of omega-3 fatty acids, known for their anti-inflammatory properties and benefits for heart health. Finally, the whole wheat bread provides dietary fiber, essential for good digestion.

"Mediterranean Dawn Bruschetta"

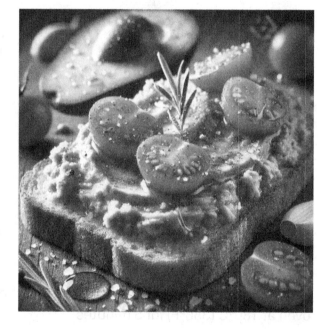

Ingredients for 2 people:

2 slices of whole wheat bread

1 ripe avocado

A handful of cherry tomatoes

1 clove of garlic

Extra virgin olive oil

Lemon juice

Salt and pepper

Procedure: Start by toasting the slices of whole wheat bread in a toaster or in the oven at 180°C (356°F) for 5 minutes.

Meanwhile, cut the avocado in half, remove the pit, and scoop out the pulp with a spoon. Place it in a bowl and mash it with a fork until creamy.

Season the avocado with lemon juice, salt, and pepper to taste. Mix well. Cut the cherry tomatoes in half or quarters, as you prefer.

Once the bread is toasted, rub one side of each slice with the garlic clove and drizzle with a bit of olive oil.

Generously spread the avocado on the bread slices, add the cherry tomatoes, and drizzle with another bit of olive oil. Add a pinch of salt and pepper to taste, if desired.

Benefits: This recipe is a nutrient-rich breakfast. Avocado is a source of monounsaturated fatty acids, beneficial for cardiovascular health and weight management. Cherry tomatoes, rich in vitamin C and lycopene, are excellent antioxidants. Finally, whole wheat bread provides fiber, contributing to satiety and intestinal health.

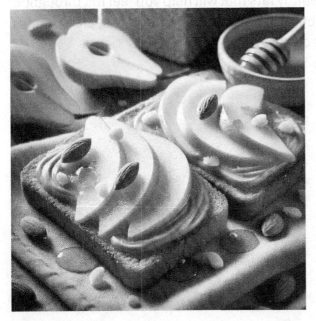

"Sweet Awakening Toast"

Ingredients for 2 people:

2 slices of gluten-free bread (or your favorite bread)

1 ripe but firm pear

1 tablespoon of almond butter or vegetable butter

A handful of nuts, chopped

Honey (optional)

If you want to make "Anti-Inflammatory Almond Butter" here's the recipe for you:

300g raw almonds

Procedure: Preheat the oven to 180°C (356°F). Spread the almonds on a baking sheet and roast in the oven for 10-12 minutes, until they become slightly golden. Let the almonds cool completely, then transfer them to a blender or food processor. Blend for 10-15 minutes, until a smooth and creamy butter forms. Store the almond butter in a sealed glass jar. Rich in vitamin E and monounsaturated fatty acids, almond butter is an excellent anti-inflammatory food.

Toast the bread until crispy and golden. Spread the almond butter on each slice of bread. Slice the pear thinly and distribute it on the bread slices. Sprinkle the chopped nuts over the pears.

If you desire an extra touch of sweetness, drizzle some honey over everything.

Benefits: Pears are an excellent source of vitamin C and fiber, essential for a healthy immune system and regular digestion. Nuts are rich in antioxidants, omega-3 fatty acids, and other nutrients that promote brain health. Additionally, almond butter is an excellent source of proteins and healthy fats that will help you feel full throughout the morning. This toast offers a perfect balance of natural sweetness, crunchiness, and creamy flavor for a tasty and invigorating wake-up.

"Frittatas and Omelettes: Start Your Day with a Zest"

"Frittata Morning Zest"

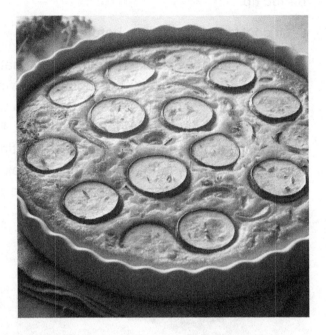

Ingredients for 2 people:

4 large eggs

1/2 cup of rice milk

1 medium zucchini

1 red bell pepper

2 tablespoons of extra virgin olive oil

A pinch of salt and pepper

1 tablespoon of fresh aromatic herbs, chopped (such as thyme, oregano, or parsley)

Procedure: Preheat the oven to 180°C (356°F) and grease a baking dish with a tablespoon of olive oil.

Thinly slice the zucchini and red bell pepper. Both zucchini and bell pepper are rich in antioxidants and fibers, essential for good digestion and to keep inflammation at bay.

Heat a tablespoon of olive oil in a pan and cook the vegetables until they become soft, which should take about 5-7 minutes.

Meanwhile, in a bowl, beat the eggs with the rice milk, aromatic herbs, salt, and pepper. The rice milk will give the frittata a creamy consistency, while the fresh herbs will add a touch of Mediterranean flavor.

Once the vegetables are ready, evenly distribute them in the greased dish; then, pour the egg mixture over them. Bake for 20-25 minutes, or until the frittata is golden and puffed up.

Let it cool for a few minutes before serving.

Benefits: "Morning Zest Frittata" is a versatile and healthy recipe that can be customized to your liking, by adding other ingredients like spinach, feta, cherry tomatoes, etc. It's rich in proteins thanks to the eggs, which help maintain satiety and provide energy throughout the morning. The vegetables, such as zucchini and bell pepper, provide fibers, vitamins, and antioxidants that support digestive health and the immune system. Additionally, the extra virgin olive oil supplies beneficial monounsaturated fats for the heart, while the aromatic herbs not only add flavor but also a variety of healthy phytochemicals.

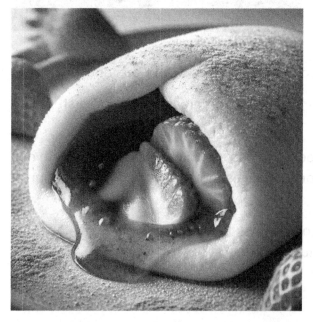

"Fruit Paradise Omelette"

Ingredients for 2 people:

4 large eggs

2 tablespoons of almond milk (or another plant-based milk of your choice)

2 tablespoons of coconut oil

4 tablespoons of sugar-free fruit jam (such as strawberry, blackberry, peach according to your taste)

A pinch of cinnamon (optional)

If you want to make the jam, here's a simple "Strawberry Jam" recipe:

500g of fresh strawberries

Juice of 1 lemon

3 tablespoons of honey

Procedure for the jam: Wash and slice the strawberries, then put them in a pot with the lemon juice and honey. Cook over low heat for about 30-40 minutes, stirring occasionally, until it reaches a spreadable consistency. Once ready, let it cool before storing it in a sterilized glass jar. This jam, sweetened with honey instead of sugar, is rich in vitamin C and antioxidants from the strawberries and lemon, ideal for an anti-inflammatory diet.

For the omelette: In a bowl, combine the eggs with almond milk. Mix until smooth.

Heat a non-stick pan over medium heat and add coconut oil.

Pour the egg and milk mixture into the pan and cook until the omelette begins to set. Spread the jam on half of the omelette and fold it in half.

Continue cooking for another minute or two, then turn off the heat and let it cool for a moment before serving. Sprinkle a pinch of cinnamon on top if you like.

Benefits: The virtues of this recipe lie in its simplicity and versatility. Eggs provide high-quality protein and good fats, while the jam offers a dose of natural sweetness. Coconut oil is known for its antibacterial and antiviral properties. Finally, almond milk offers a healthy plant-based drink rich in vitamin E, a fat-soluble vitamin that acts as a powerful antioxidant in the body. Together, these ingredients create a delicious and healthy omelette that will start your day off on the right foot.

"Green Aroma Frittata"

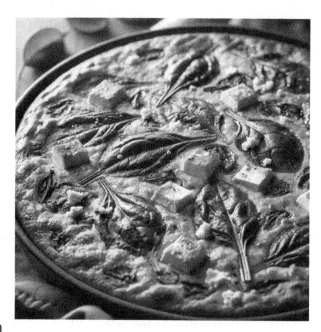

Ingredients for 2 people:

4 large eggs

4 handfuls of fresh spinach

100 grams of feta cheese

2 tablespoons of olive oil

Salt and pepper to taste

Procedure: Heat the olive oil in a non-stick pan over medium heat.

Add the spinach and cook until wilted, about 2-3 minutes.

In the meantime, beat the eggs in a bowl. Add crumbled feta, salt, and pepper.

Pour the egg mixture over the spinach in the pan, reduce the heat to low, cover, and cook until the omelette is set, about 5 minutes. With a spatula, flip the omelette and cook for another 2-3 minutes.

Benefits: This spinach and feta frittata is a nutritious breakfast option that offers a good dose of protein from the eggs and feta, while the spinach adds a healthy dose of vitamin K, vitamin A, and iron. Together, they create a delicious and well-balanced meal that will give you energy throughout the morning.

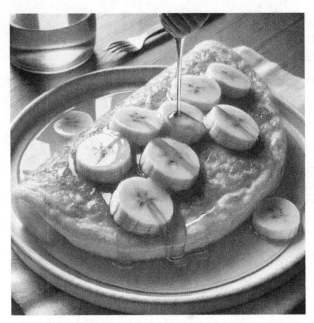

"Golden Awakening: Banana Omelette with Maple Syrup"

Ingredients for 2 people:

4 eggs

2 ripe bananas

2 tablespoons of maple syrup

2 tablespoons of coconut oil

Procedure: Beat the eggs in a bowl until they become frothy. Heat the coconut oil in a non-stick pan over medium heat.

Pour the beaten eggs into the hot pan, making sure they evenly cover the surface.

As the omelette begins to cook, slice the banana and distribute it evenly over the surface.

When the omelette is halfway done, fold it in half with a spatula. Cook for another minute, then transfer the omelette onto a plate. Drizzle with maple syrup.

Benefits: This "Golden Awakening" recipe offers a tasty way to start the day. Eggs provide high-quality protein to support muscles and maintain satiety, while bananas are rich in fiber and potassium for heart health. Coconut oil adds a touch of tropical flavor and provides medium-chain fatty acids for lasting energy. Finally, the maple syrup gives a sweet finishing touch, supplying important minerals like manganese and zinc. Waking up has never been so sweet and healthy.

Quote: *"Salad is the art of presenting nature on a plate." - Julia Child.*

CHAPTER 9

"Simple but Tasty Salads and Side Dishes"

Rediscovering side dishes and salads in today's cuisine reveals a journey rich in surprising flavors, a sensory spectacle that goes beyond the simple function of 'accompaniment'. Like an explorer diving into uncharted territories, we discover that these dishes too can transform into undisputed protagonists of the table.

Imagine vibrant salads that soar beyond the role of mere 'green aggregate'. Consider side dishes shedding their cloak of modesty to reveal themselves as authentic triumphs of creativity and flavor. The freshness of a summer salad releases the scents of the field, while winter sides evoke the warmth of the fireplace and family laughter.

In our journey, we discover the wonder of contrasts, a sweet call wrapped in the poignant emotion of surprise, or the rustle of tenacity dancing with the caress of tenderness.

Thus, with a dash of creativity and a love for exploration, these 'simple' dishes elevate to new heights, transforming into a culinary experience that touches the soul and delights the palate. Venture with us in this exploration of sides and salads, a journey that will grant you a newfound appreciation for the beauty and goodness of these too often underestimated dishes.

"The Magic Salads"

"Summer Salad in Pink: Mixed salad, Turkey, Strawberries, and Balsamic Vinegar"

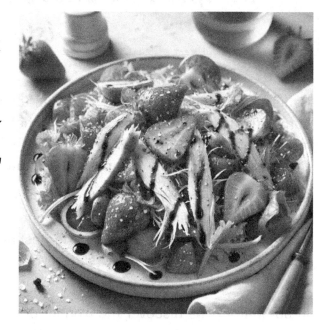

Ingredients for 4 people:

200g mixed salad

400g turkey

250g fresh strawberries

Balsamic vinegar to taste

Extra virgin olive oil

Salt and pepper to taste

Procedure: Start with preparing the turkey strips. Cut the turkey into thin strips and sauté in a pan with a drizzle of extra virgin olive oil until golden. Once cooked, let cool.

While the turkey cools, wash the mixed salad and arrange them on the serving dish. The mixed salad, with their varied colors and crunchy texture, form the ideal bed for the following ingredients.

Wash the strawberries, dry them, and slice them thinly. Add them to the mixed salad. The strawberries will add a touch of sweetness and color to the dish, creating a beautiful contrast with the vegetables and turkey.

When the turkey has cooled, shred it by hand and arrange it on the salad. Finally, dress the salad with a drizzle of extra virgin olive oil, balsamic vinegar, salt, and pepper.

The recipe is ready! A simple and refined dish, perfect for a summer lunch or a light dinner. The flavors are balanced: the sweetness of the strawberries contrasts with the savoriness of the turkey, and the balsamic vinegar adds a touch of acidity that balances everything out.

Benefits: The nutritional properties of this salad are remarkable: turkey is a source of lean protein, strawberries are rich in antioxidants and vitamin C, and mixed greens are a source of fiber and vitamins. A delicious and nutritious dish, perfect for those following an anti-inflammatory diet.

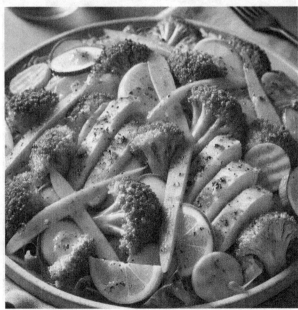

"Radiant Broccoli, Chicken, and Carrot Salad"

Ingredients for 4 people:

1 large broccoli

2 chicken breasts

2 large carrots

2 tablespoons of extra virgin olive oil

Juice of 1 lemon

1 teaspoon of turmeric

Salt and pepper to taste

Procedure: Start by cutting the broccoli into florets and julienning the carrots. Steam both until they are tender but still crisp. Meanwhile, grill or pan-fry the chicken breasts with a drizzle of oil until golden, then slice them into thin strips.

In a large bowl, combine the broccoli, carrots, and chicken. In a separate small bowl, mix the oil, lemon juice, turmeric, salt, and pepper to create a dressing. Pour the dressing over the salad and mix well to combine all the ingredients.

Benefits: "Radiant Broccoli, Chicken, and Carrot Salad" is a complete meal, rich in proteins thanks to the chicken, and vitamins and fibers provided by broccoli and carrots. The turmeric-based dressing adds a spicy and beneficial touch, thanks to the anti-inflammatory properties of this spice. A tasty and healthy choice for a light lunch or dinner.

"Green Forest Salad"

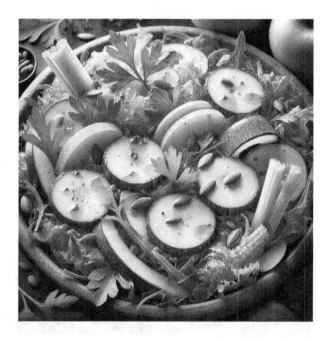

Ingredients for 4 people:

2 bunches of arugula

2 bunches of fresh parsley

4 stalks of celery

4 zucchinis

2 green apples

2 lemons

4 tablespoons of extra virgin olive oil

Pumpkin and sunflower seeds to taste

Salt and black pepper to taste

Procedure: Thoroughly wash all ingredients. Slice the zucchinis and celery into thin rounds. Cut the apple into thin slices, keeping the skin on for an extra fiber boost. Chop the parsley and add it to the arugula in a large bowl. Add the sliced vegetables and apple.

Dress with extra virgin olive oil, the juice of one lemon, salt, and pepper. Mix well and finish with a handful of pumpkin and sunflower seeds.

Benefits: "Green Forest" is an explosion of freshness and benefits. The vegetables, fruit, and parsley, rich in vitamins C and K, pumpkin seeds with magnesium and zinc, and green apple with vitamins A and C, help to balance the intestinal flora and keep the body alkaline. Extra virgin olive oil provides heart-healthy fatty acids. A dish that's pure well-being!

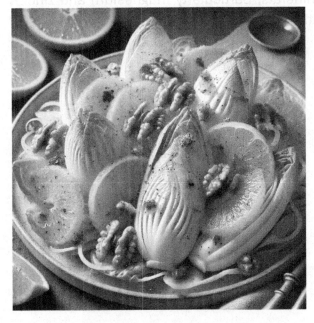

"Belgian Endive Salad with Oranges and Caramelized Nuts"

Ingredients for 4 people:

4 heads of Belgian endive

2 oranges

150g of walnuts

2 tablespoons of honey

4 tablespoons of extra virgin olive oil

1 tablespoon of balsamic vinegar

Salt and black pepper to taste

Procedure: Preheat the oven to 180°C (356°F). Place the walnuts on a baking sheet lined with parchment paper and drizzle with honey. Bake for 10-15 minutes, or until the nuts are caramelized and crunchy. Let cool.

Wash and dry the Belgian endive and cut it into strips. Peel the oranges and slice them thinly.

Prepare the dressing by mixing the olive oil, balsamic vinegar, salt, and pepper.

Arrange the Belgian endive and orange slices on a serving plate. Sprinkle with the caramelized nuts and dress with the vinaigrette.

Benefits: This salad is a true concentration of nutrients. Belgian endive is rich in vitamin K and vitamin A, useful for bone and vision health. Oranges provide an excellent dose of vitamin C, a powerful antioxidant. Finally, the caramelized nuts provide proteins, healthy fats, and minerals, particularly magnesium and zinc. A tasty and beneficial dish for your health!

"Autumn Forest Salad"

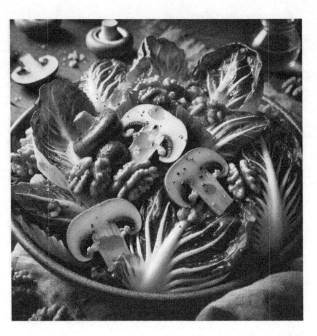

Ingredients for 4 people:

2 heads of radicchio

400 grams of champignon mushrooms

2 oranges

4 tablespoons of extra virgin olive oil

Himalayan pink salt and black pepper to taste

A handful of shelled walnuts

2 cloves of garlic

Procedure: Start by washing and slicing the radicchio into strips and the mushrooms into thin slices. Heat a drizzle of olive oil in a pan, add the peeled garlic and mushrooms, and sauté over medium heat for 5 minutes. Remove the garlic, add the radicchio, and continue cooking for another 5 minutes. Turn off the heat and let it cool slightly.

In the meantime, prepare a dressing with the oil, orange juice, salt, and pepper. Place the radicchio and mushrooms in a bowl, dress with the emulsion, and finish with crumbled walnuts.

Benefits: The "Autumn Forest" dish combines the vitamin K from radicchio, selenium and potassium from mushrooms, vitamin C from oranges, and omega-3 from walnuts. This mix, along with the extra virgin olive oil, provides anti-inflammatory benefits and supports heart health. A dish that is a real treat for both the palate and well-being!

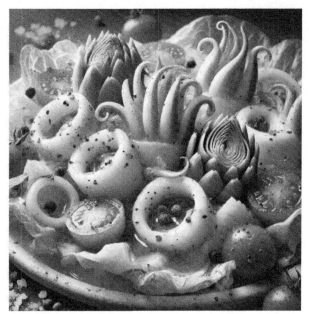

"Sea Fantasy Salad: Baby Squids, Artichokes, and Tomatoes on a Bed of Iceberg"

Ingredients for 4 people:

400 g of fresh baby squids

2 large artichokes

200 g of cherry tomatoes

1 iceberg lettuce

Juice of 1 lemon

2 cloves of garlic

Extra virgin olive oil

Salt and pepper to taste

Procedure: Begin with cleaning the baby squids, a task that can be made enjoyable by the anticipation of the flavors you are about to create. Once cleaned, briefly sauté the baby squids in a pan with a drizzle of oil and garlic until they become translucent.

Separately, clean the artichokes by removing the tougher outer leaves and cutting them in half. Immerse them in water with lemon juice to prevent them from blackening. Then, slice the artichokes thinly and sauté in a pan with a drizzle of oil until they become tender.

Cut the cherry tomatoes in half and gently squeeze to remove the seeds. Add them to the pan with the artichokes for just a couple of minutes, just enough to warm them up.

At this point, prepare the bed of iceberg lettuce in a large bowl, place the baby squids, artichokes, and tomatoes on top. Dress with extra virgin olive oil, salt, and pepper to taste.

Enjoy the salad immediately or store it in the refrigerator for an hour for a tasty cold dish.

Benefits: This recipe is a hymn to health: baby squids are rich in proteins and Omega-3, artichokes are known for their detoxifying properties, tomatoes are a source of lycopene, a powerful antioxidant, and the iceberg lettuce adds freshness and fiber. An explosion of flavor and well-being in every bite!

"Sea Breeze: A Whiff of the Sea on Your Plate."

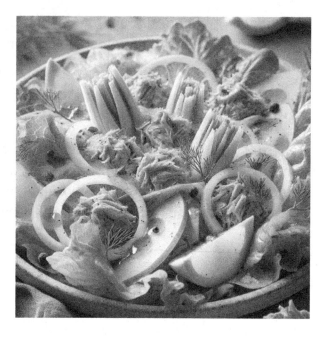

Ingredients for 4 people:

4 heads of lettuce

2 large fennels

200 grams of natural tuna

2 green apples

4 tablespoons of extra virgin olive oil

Juice of 2 lemons, salt, and pepper to taste

Procedure: Start by washing and drying the lettuce. Clean the fennels, remove the core, and slice them thinly. Drain the tuna and flake it. Wash the apples, remove the core, and slice them thinly.

In a large bowl, combine the lettuce, fennel, tuna, and apples. Prepare a dressing with the oil, lemon juice, salt, and pepper. Pour the dressing over the salad and mix gently.

Benefits: This recipe, "Sea Breeze," offers an excellent combination of anti-inflammatory ingredients such as fennel, rich in vitamin C, and tuna, a source of Omega-3. The lettuce and apple, finally, contribute to providing fiber, essential for the well-being of the digestive system. A dish that, besides being an explosion of taste, is also light and nutritious, contributing to keeping the body in shape and strengthening the immune system.

"Delicious Side Dishes"

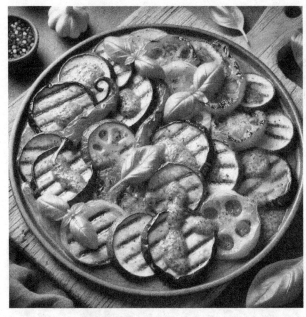

"Mediterranean Flavor of Baked and Grilled Vegetables with Basil Sauce"

Ingredients for 4 people:

4 medium eggplants

4 zucchinis

4 bell peppers, two red and two yellow

4 tablespoons of extra virgin olive oil

Salt and pepper to taste

For the basil sauce:

2 bunches of fresh basil

200ml of extra virgin olive oil

2 cloves of garlic

Salt and pepper to taste

Procedure: Begin by preheating the oven to 180 degrees Celsius. Slice the eggplants into thick slices, sprinkle them with some salt, and let them rest for 15 minutes. Meanwhile, slice the zucchinis into thin slices and the bell peppers into strips. Rinse the eggplants to remove excess salt and dry them. Place all the vegetables on a baking tray, season with olive oil, salt, and pepper, then bake for 20-25 minutes or until tender and golden.

For the sauce, blend the basil, garlic, and olive oil in a blender until smooth. Taste and adjust for salt and pepper.

Serve the vegetables warm or at room temperature, topped with a spoonful of basil sauce. You can also grill the vegetables for a smokier flavor.

Benefits: The vegetables, rich in vitamins and antioxidants, are cooked in a way that preserves most of their nutrients. The basil sauce, with its content of olive oil, provides good fats that help reduce inflammation. A side dish that delights the palate and benefits the body.

"Baked Vegetables with Herb Breadcrumbs"

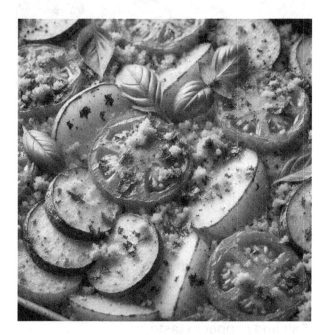

Ingredients for 4 people:

4 medium potatoes

8 ripe tomatoes

200g of breadcrumbs

4 cloves of garlic

2 bunches of fresh parsley

2 bunches of fresh basil

4 tablespoons of extra virgin olive oil

Salt and pepper to taste

Procedure: Preheat the oven to 200°C. Meanwhile, slice the potatoes and tomatoes into thick slices, about 1 cm thick. Arrange the slices on a baking tray lined with parchment paper, alternating potatoes, and tomatoes.

In a blender, combine the breadcrumbs, garlic, parsley, basil, olive oil, salt, and pepper. Blend until you get an herb breadcrumb mixture. Spread this breadcrumb mixture over the potato and tomato slices, pressing gently with your hands to make it stick.

Bake for 30-35 minutes, or until the vegetables are tender and the breadcrumbs are golden. Serve the baked vegetable dish hot, directly from the tray.

Benefits: "Baked Vegetables with Herb Breadcrumbs" is a dish rich in flavors and nutrition. Potatoes and tomatoes are a good source of vitamins, minerals, and fibers, which help keep the body healthy. The herb breadcrumbs, with their content of olive oil, provide good fats and antioxidants, useful for fighting inflammation. A simple and tasty side dish that is good for both the palate and the body.

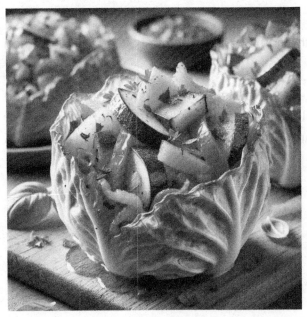

"Crunchy Cabbage Baskets with Sautéed Vegetables"

Ingredients for 4 people:

For the baskets:

8 large cabbage leaves

2 tablespoons of olive oil

Salt and pepper to taste

For the filling:

1 red bell pepper, diced

1 yellow bell pepper, diced

2 medium zucchinis, diced

2 medium carrots, diced

1 red onion, chopped

2 tablespoons of olive oil

Salt and pepper to taste

Fresh herbs for garnishing (parsley, basil, thyme)

Procedure: Preheat the oven to 180°C. Arrange the cabbage leaves on a baking sheet lined with parchment paper. Brush each leaf with a bit of olive oil and sprinkle with salt and pepper. Bake for 10-15 minutes, or until the leaves are crispy.

Meanwhile, prepare the filling. In a large pan, heat the olive oil. Add the onion and sauté until translucent. Add the bell peppers, zucchinis, and carrots. Cook over medium heat for about 10 minutes, or until the vegetables are tender. Season with salt and pepper.

Fill each crispy cabbage basket with the sautéed vegetable mix. Garnish with fresh herbs before serving.

Benefits: These crispy cabbage baskets are a dish rich in vitamins, minerals, and fibers thanks to the variety of vegetables used. Cabbage, in particular, is known for its high content of vitamin K, which contributes to bone health and blood clotting. A delicious and nutritious dish!

"Baked Pumpkin and Kale with Turmeric"

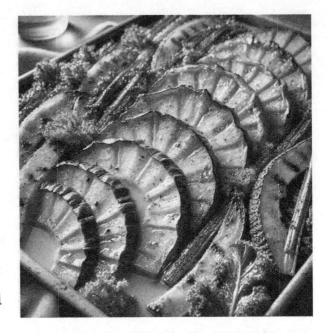

Ingredients for 4 people:

2 small pumpkins

400g of kale

2 teaspoons of turmeric powder

4 tablespoons of extra virgin olive oil

Salt and pepper to taste

Procedure: Preheat the oven to 200°C. Cut the pumpkin into slices after removing the seeds and skin. Clean the kale by removing the tough central part and cutting it into strips. Arrange the pumpkin and kale on a baking tray lined with parchment paper.

In a bowl, mix the extra virgin olive oil with turmeric, a pinch of salt, and pepper. Brush this dressing over the vegetables, trying to distribute it evenly.

Bake for 20-25 minutes, or until the vegetables are tender and slightly caramelized. Serve the pumpkin and kale warm, possibly with a drizzle of raw olive oil.

Benefits: A dish rich in antioxidants and fiber, thanks to the presence of pumpkin and kale. Turmeric, with its anti-inflammatory and antioxidant properties, adds an extra touch of flavor and well-being. A colorful and healthy start to a meal, perfect for the autumn season.

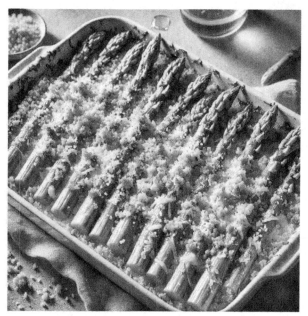

"Gratinated Asparagus with Whole Wheat Bread and Lactose-Free Cheese"

Ingredients for 4 people:

4 bunches of asparagus

200g of whole wheat dry bread

200g of lactose-free cheese

4 tablespoons of extra virgin olive oil

Salt and pepper to taste

Procedure: Preheat the oven to 200°C (392°F). Clean the asparagus by removing the hard end of the stem and arrange them in a baking dish. In a mixer, grind the dry bread until you get a coarse breadcrumb. Add the lactose-free cheese cut into pieces and grind again until you get a homogeneous mixture.

Spread this bread and cheese mixture over the asparagus, pressing it down slightly with your hands to make it stick. Drizzle everything with extra virgin olive oil, then add a pinch of salt and pepper.

Bake for 15-20 minutes, or until the topping is golden and crispy. Serve the gratinated asparagus hot to best appreciate the contrast between the softness of the asparagus and the crunchiness of the gratin.

Benefits: This dish is rich in fibers and antioxidants, thanks to the asparagus. The lactose-free cheese makes it digestible even for those with lactose intolerance, while the whole wheat bread provides additional fibers and satiety. A simple, yet tasty and nutritious dish, perfect for starting a meal in a healthy way

Quote: *"Good food is the foundation of genuine happiness." - Auguste Escoffier.*

CHAPTER 10

"Glorious and Nutritious Warm or Cold First Courses"

Imagine walking through a lush forest, the sounds of nature lulling you, and the air soaked in tranquility. Thinking of warm first courses is like feeling the comforting embrace of the forest: pasta, flexible and sturdy like the roots of trees; gnocchi, small earthy gems hidden under the foliage; lasagnas, layered like the complexity of the ecosystem; risottos, slow and calm like the growth of vegetation; soups, nourishment flowing like the streams that cross the ground.

On the other hand, thinking of cold dishes is like observing an open field under the blue sky. There's the freshness of grain bowls, like the wind whispering through the ears of grain; cold pastas, quick and versatile like hares running through the meadows; poke, a rainbow of flavors like wildflowers dotting the countryside.

In every dish, whether warm or cold, it is possible to rediscover the essence of nature, a celebration of life that blooms in every bite. As we walk this gastronomic path, we are called to reflect, to connect with the depth of our roots, and to live with the lightness of a butterfly's wings. Let us enter this world with curiosity and joy, ready to discover how nature can nourish us in every aspect of our life.

"Hot Dishes that Warm Body and Spirit"
"The Timeless Pleasure of Pasta"

"Penne with Forest Flavors: A Meeting of Past and Future"

Ingredients for 4 people:

400 g of whole wheat penne pasta

400 g of mixed mushrooms

2 cloves of garlic

4 tablespoons of extra virgin olive oil

Salt and pepper to taste

2 handfuls of fresh parsley

2 teaspoons of turmeric powder

Procedure: Cook the pasta in plenty of salted water until al dente. Meanwhile, clean the mushrooms and slice them thinly. In a non-stick pan, heat the oil and add the peeled garlic cloves. When the garlic is golden, add the mushrooms. Cook over medium heat for 10-15 minutes, until the mushrooms are golden. Add the turmeric and mix well.

Drain the pasta and transfer it to the pan with the mushrooms. Mix well to absorb the flavor. Adjust with salt and pepper, and sprinkle with chopped fresh parsley before serving.

Benefits: The "Penne with Forest Flavors" are a true delight for the palate, enriched with mushrooms and turmeric that, in addition to providing flavor, have anti-inflammatory properties. A simple, tasty, and healthy recipe that pays homage to Italian tradition, with a touch of innovation.

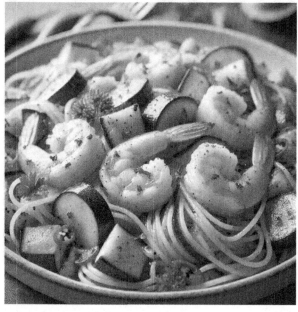

"Spaghetti Elegance: A Dance of Flavor and Health"

Ingredients for 4 people:

400g of gluten-free spaghetti

4 tablespoons of extra virgin olive oil

2 cloves of garlic

1 fresh red chili pepper

2 bunches of fresh parsley

400g of cleaned shrimp

2 medium zucchinis

Salt and black pepper to taste

Procedure: Bring a pot of water to a boil for the pasta. Meanwhile, wash and cube the zucchini. In a large pan, heat the oil and add the crushed garlic and chopped chili pepper. Sauté for a couple of minutes, then add the shrimp and zucchini. Sauté over medium heat for 5-7 minutes.

Meanwhile, cook the spaghetti according to the package instructions. Once cooked, drain them and transfer to the pan with the shrimp and zucchini. Add the chopped parsley, adjust with salt, and pepper, and mix well to blend the flavors.

Benefits: The "Spaghetti Elegance" offers a perfect balance between taste and nutritional benefits. Olive oil, garlic, chili pepper, and zucchini have anti-inflammatory properties. The shrimp provide high-quality protein. This elegant and nutritious recipe is a true homage to the Mediterranean diet, surprising the palate without compromising on health.

"Autumn Fusilli: A Hug of Well-Being"

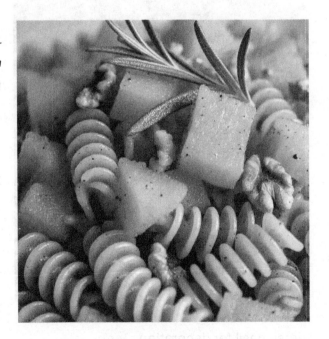

Ingredients for 4 people:

400g of spelt fusilli

4 tablespoons of extra virgin olive oil

2 cloves of garlic

400g of pumpkin

2 sprigs of rosemary

100g of walnuts

Salt and black pepper to taste

Procedure: Begin by cutting the pumpkin into cubes. In a pan, heat the oil and add the crushed garlic and rosemary. After a couple of minutes, add the pumpkin and cook over medium heat for about 15 minutes, or until softened.

Meanwhile, bring a pot of water to a boil and cook the fusilli according to the package instructions. Drain the pasta al dente and transfer it to the pan with the pumpkin. Add the chopped walnuts, adjust with salt, and pepper, and mix well.

Benefits: This pasta represents a perfect marriage between taste and nutrition. The pumpkin, with its sweet flavor, is rich in vitamins A and C, both antioxidants. The walnuts provide Omega-3s, known for their anti-inflammatory properties. Finally, spelt pasta is an excellent source of fiber. This recipe is a true tribute to autumn, combining its distinctive flavors with the desire to eat healthily and balanced.

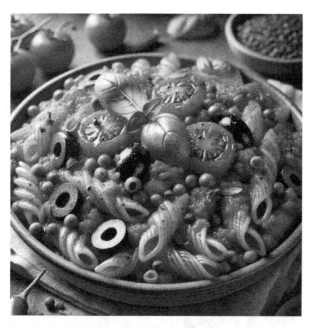

"Red Lentil Pasta"

Ingredients for 4 people:

400g of red lentil pasta

2 tablespoons of extra virgin olive oil

2 cloves of garlic

1 red chili pepper

500g of peeled tomatoes

100g of pitted black olives

Salt and black pepper to taste

Fresh basil for decoration

Procedure: Start by heating the oil in a pan and adding the crushed garlic and chopped chili pepper. After a couple of minutes, add the peeled tomatoes and black olives, then season with salt and pepper. Cook over medium heat for about 20 minutes, or until the sauce has thickened.

Meanwhile, bring a pot of water to a boil and cook the red lentil pasta according to the package instructions. Once cooked, drain the pasta, and transfer it to the pan with the sauce. Mix well to coat the pasta.

Serve the pasta hot, garnishing with fresh basil leaves.

Benefits: This dish combines the nutritional benefits of red lentils, rich in protein and fiber, with those of tomatoes, rich in vitamin C and lycopene, a powerful antioxidant. The black olives contribute healthy fats and vitamin E. The result is a balanced, nutritious, and flavorful dish!

"Purple Maccheroncini"

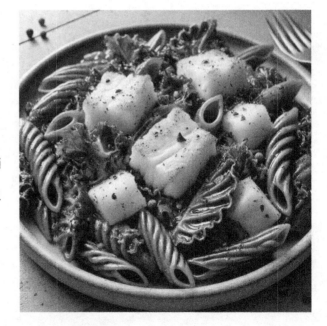

Ingredients for 4 people:

400g of whole wheat maccheroncini

4 tablespoons of extra virgin olive oil

2 cloves of garlic

400g of cod

2 bunches of purple cabbage

Salt and black pepper to taste

Procedure: Start by boiling the purple cabbage until it becomes soft. Transfer it to a blender and blend until you get a smooth cream.

In a pan, heat the oil and add the crushed garlic. Once golden, add the diced cod and cook over medium heat until it turns white.

Meanwhile, cook the maccheroncini in boiling salted water following the package instructions. Drain them al dente and add the purple cabbage cream. Mix well and add the cod. Season with salt and pepper to taste.

Benefits: "Purple Maccheroncini" is an explosion of flavors and colors. The purple cabbage cream, besides giving an amazing color, is rich in antioxidants, while the cod provides high-quality proteins and Omega-3. A dish that combines the delicate taste of the sea with the boldness of vegetables for an unforgettable culinary experience.

"Unbeatable Gnocchi"

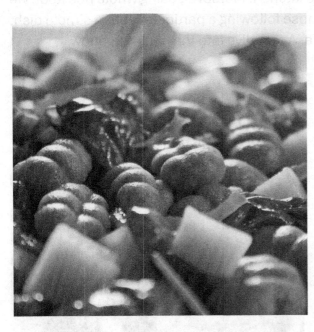

"The Gnocchi: Rainbow of Health"

Ingredients for 4 people:

For the gnocchi:

800g of purple potatoes

200g of whole rice flour

Salt to taste

For the dressing:

100g of red cabbage

100g of fresh spinach

100g of yellow squash

Extra virgin olive oil

Salt and pepper to taste

Procedure: Boil the potatoes in salted water until they are tender. Mash them in a bowl and let cool. Add the rice flour and salt, work until you have a smooth dough.

Form cylinders of dough and cut them into small gnocchi. Cook the gnocchi in boiling salted water until they float, then drain them.

For the dressings, cut the red cabbage, spinach, and squash into small pieces. Sauté each in a pan with a bit of oil, salt, and pepper.

Finally, dress the gnocchi with the sautéed vegetables. Serve hot.

Benefits: A colorful and nutritious recipe, rich in antioxidants thanks to the red cabbage, spinach, and squash. A creative dish, full of fibers, vitamins, and minerals that perfectly reflects innovation in the kitchen. Moreover, using whole rice flour, we obtain gluten-free gnocchi, ideal for those following a particular diet. A simple dish, yet surprising in flavor and appearance. A true dive into the health rainbow.

"Gnocchi: Ruby Reflections on the Table"

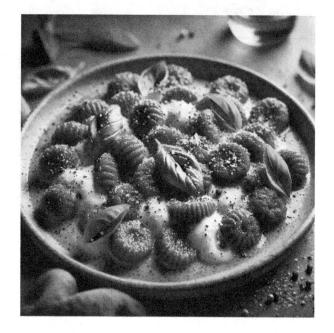

Ingredients for 4 people:

500g of red potatoes

200g of flour

1 medium beetroot

1 teaspoon of salt

150g of ricotta

100g of grated Parmesan cheese

2 tablespoons of extra virgin olive oil

Black pepper to taste

Fresh basil leaves as needed

Procedure: First, boil the potatoes and beetroot in boiling water until they are soft. Drain and let cool, then peel and mash them.

Add the flour and salt, and knead until you have a smooth dough. Form cylinders of dough and cut the gnocchi.

For the dressing, mix the ricotta with the Parmesan, olive oil, and black pepper. Cook the gnocchi in boiling salted water until they float to the surface, then drain and dress them with the cheese cream. Add fresh basil leaves to taste before serving.

Benefits: These gnocchi not only offer an unmistakable taste but also a remarkable visual impact. The high concentration of antioxidants and the anti-inflammatory effect of beetroot and red potatoes make this dish nutritious and beneficial for health, helping to keep the body healthy and fight inflammation.

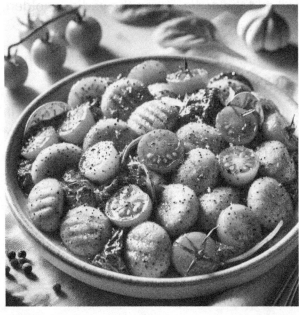

"Green Gnocchi: A Revolutionary Culinary Experience"

Ingredients for 4 people:

For the gnocchi:

500 g of potatoes

200 g of fresh spinach

200 g of flour

1 egg

Salt to taste

For the dressing:

1 clove of garlic

200 g of cherry tomatoes

2 tablespoons of extra virgin olive oil

Salt and pepper to taste

Procedure: Start with the gnocchi. Boil the potatoes until soft. Meanwhile, wash the spinach and briefly boil it in boiling water. Drain the spinach and once cool enough to handle, squeeze out the excess water.

Mash the potatoes and spinach in a bowl, gradually adding the flour and a pinch of salt. Add the egg and knead until you have a uniform mixture. Form cylinders of dough and cut the gnocchi.

For the dressing, heat the oil in a pan and add the garlic. When the garlic is golden, add the halved cherry tomatoes, season with salt and pepper.

Boil the gnocchi in salted water until they float. Drain the gnocchi and add them to the dressing in the pan. Gently mix to combine.

Benefits: The essence of this recipe lies in the presence of spinach, rich in antioxidants and anti-inflammatory agents, and cherry tomatoes, a source of lycopene, a powerful antioxidant. A delicious and beneficial dish!

"Colorful Euphoria Gnocchi"

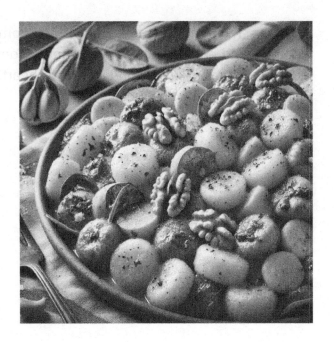

Ingredients for 4 people:

For the gnocchi:

600g of potatoes

200g of spinach

2 medium carrots

200g of flour

1 egg yolk

Salt to taste

For the dressing:

2 cloves of garlic

Extra virgin olive oil

100g of walnuts

Salt and pepper to taste

Procedure: Begin by boiling the potatoes and carrots with their skin on until soft. In parallel, cook the spinach. Once cooked, combine them with the potatoes and carrots in a mixer, blending everything until a smooth cream is obtained.

Once cooled, add the egg yolk, flour, and a pinch of salt to the mixture, working the dough until it achieves a soft and non-sticky consistency. From there, form cylinders and cut the gnocchi.

For the dressing, fry the garlic in oil in a pan, add the chopped walnuts, and let them brown for a few minutes. Once the gnocchi are cooked, drain them, and add them to the dressing in the pan. Gently stir and season with salt and pepper.

Benefits: A burst of well-being emanates from this dish: spinach and carrots bring vitamins and antioxidants, while walnuts contribute essential fatty acids that are anti-inflammatory and good for the heart. A true embrace of health and deliciousness for the palate.

"Risottos: Every Grain a Delight"

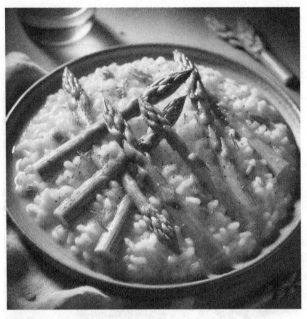

"Rainbow Risotto: An Explosion of Asparagus and Saffron"

Ingredients for 4 people:

350g of Carnaroli rice

1 bunch of fresh asparagus

1 sachet of saffron

1 white onion

1 liter of vegetable broth

Salt and pepper to taste

Extra virgin olive oil

Procedure: Start by cleaning and cutting the asparagus, reserving the tips. In a saucepan, sauté the chopped onion with a drizzle of oil. Add the asparagus (except for the tips) and let them flavor. Add the rice and toast it for a couple of minutes.

Begin to add the broth a little at a time, waiting for the rice to absorb it before adding the next ladle. Midway through cooking, add the saffron to give the characteristic golden color.

Continue cooking by adding the broth and, in the last minute, add the asparagus tips. Season with salt and pepper, and your risotto is ready to be served.

Benefits: "The Rainbow Risotto" combines asparagus, rich in vitamins A, C, E, and saffron, a natural anti-inflammatory. The pairing offers a tasty, colorful, and beneficial dish for the body.

"Brilliant Black Risotto: A Symphony of Artichokes and Vegetables"

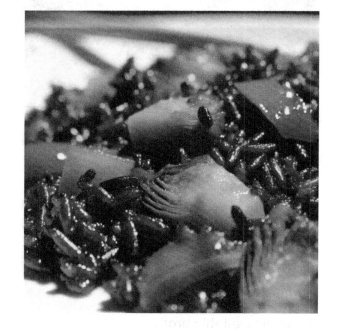

Ingredients for 4 people:

350g of Venere rice

4 fresh artichokes

1 red bell pepper

1 red onion

1 liter of vegetable broth

Salt and pepper to taste

Extra virgin olive oil

Procedure: Start by cleaning and slicing the artichokes and bell pepper, set them aside. In a large saucepan, sauté the chopped onion with a drizzle of oil. Add the artichokes and bell pepper, let them flavor for a few minutes.

Add the Venere rice and toast it for a couple of minutes. Begin to pour in the broth gradually, allowing the rice to absorb it before adding the next ladle. Continue cooking until the rice is al dente.

Adjust with salt and pepper, and your Brilliant Black Risotto is ready to be served, a true explosion of flavors with every bite!

Benefits: A dish rich in vitamins and minerals, thanks to the presence of artichokes, bell peppers, and Venere rice. Artichokes are an excellent anti-inflammatory and source of vitamin C, while Venere rice provides fiber and antioxidants. A balanced recipe that pleases the palate and nourishes the body.

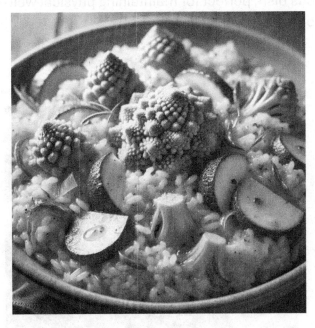

"Vegetable Harmony Risotto"

Ingredients for 4 people:

350g of whole grain rice

2 zucchinis

1 bunch of Romanesco broccoli

1 red onion

2 cloves of garlic

1.5 liters of vegetable broth

1 teaspoon of turmeric

2 tablespoons of olive oil

Salt and pepper to taste

Procedure: Start by chopping the onion and garlic, then sauté them in a large pan with olive oil. Meanwhile, dice the zucchinis and separate the Romanesco broccoli florets. Add the vegetables to the pan and cook for 5 minutes.

Now, add the rice and turmeric, mix well so the rice is flavored. Begin to add the vegetable broth one ladle at a time, stirring occasionally. Cook the risotto for about 20-25 minutes, until the rice is al dente, and the broth is completely absorbed. Season with salt and pepper and serve immediately.

Benefits: "Vegetable Harmony Risotto" is a dish that combines the rustic taste of whole grain rice with the sweetness of the vegetables, enriched with turmeric, known for its anti-inflammatory properties. It is a creamy, flavorful dish, rich in fibers and vitamins, especially vitamins A and C, precious for the immune system and skin health. A balanced, tasty, and nutritious dish, perfect for maintaining physical well-being without giving up the pleasure of taste.

"Bright Purple Risotto"

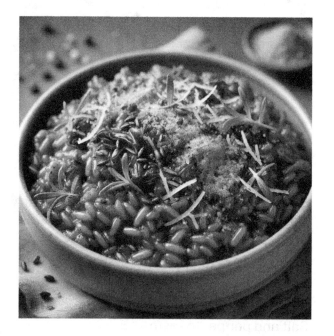

Ingredients for 4 people:

350g of Carnaroli rice

200g of red cabbage

1 white onion

1.5 liters of vegetable broth

100g of Parmesan cheese

2 tablespoons of extra virgin olive oil

Salt and pepper to taste

1 teaspoon of turmeric

1 teaspoon of cumin

Procedure: Start by chopping the onion and cook it over medium heat in a pan with the oil. Meanwhile, finely chop the red cabbage and add it to the pan. Add turmeric and cumin, then mix well. Now, add the rice and let it toast for a few minutes, then begin to add the broth, one ladle at a time, stirring occasionally. Continue to cook the risotto for 18-20 minutes, until the rice is al dente. Season with salt and pepper, turn off the heat, and stir in the Parmesan cheese. Let it rest for a couple of minutes and then serve.

Benefits: A dish rich in antioxidants, thanks to the red cabbage, which also gives a splendid purple color to the rice. Turmeric and cumin add a spicy note and are known for their anti-inflammatory properties. It is a risotto with an intense taste, rich in vitamins A, C, K, and fibers, thanks to the use of red cabbage and whole grain rice. A dish that combines well-being and the pleasure of taste.

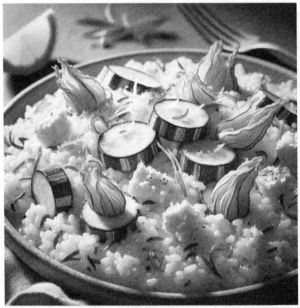

"Elegant Risotto: Zucchini Flowers and Goat Cheese"

Ingredients for 4 people:

350g of whole grain rice

12 zucchini flowers

150g of fresh goat cheese

1 white onion

1.5 liters of vegetable broth

2 tablespoons of extra virgin olive oil

Salt and pepper to taste

Grated zest of 1 lemon

Procedure: Start by chopping the onion and cooking it over medium heat in a pan with the oil. Clean the zucchini flowers, removing the internal pistil and cutting them into strips. Add the zucchini flowers to the pan and cook for a couple of minutes.

Now, add the rice and let it toast for a few minutes, then start adding the broth, one ladle at a time, stirring occasionally. Continue to cook the risotto for 18-20 minutes, until the rice is al dente.

Turn off the heat, add the goat cheese in pieces, and stir until it has completely melted. Season with salt and pepper, then add the grated lemon zest. Let it rest for a couple of minutes before serving.

Benefits: This risotto is a true concentrate of flavors and health benefits. Zucchini flowers are known for their diuretic and anti-inflammatory properties, while goat cheese is more digestible compared to other cheeses and rich in calcium. The lemon zest, in addition to giving a touch of freshness to the dish, is rich in antioxidants. The result is a delicate dish, but full of taste and nutrients.

"Lasagne: Stop Feeling Guilty"

"Greenleaf Lasagna: The Vegetarian Embrace that Nourishes Body and Soul"

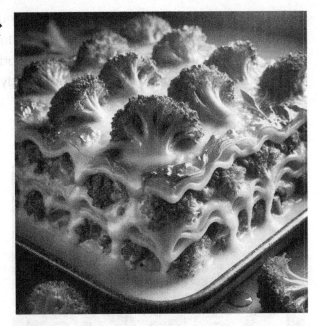

Ingredients for 4 people:

12 lasagna sheets

1 large broccoli

500 ml of béchamel sauce (made with oat milk)

50 g of rice flour

50 g of vegetable margarine

Salt and pepper to taste

Nutmeg to taste

EVO oil

Procedure: Begin by cleaning the broccoli and dividing it into florets, then boil it in salted water for 10 minutes. Drain and let cool. Prepare the béchamel: in a saucepan, melt the margarine, add the flour, and stir for a couple of minutes. Slowly pour in the oat milk, continuing to stir to avoid lumps. Add salt, pepper, and a sprinkle of nutmeg. Cook for about 10 minutes until you obtain a soft and velvety cream.

Preheat the oven to 180 degrees. Oil a baking dish and arrange a first layer of lasagna sheets, cover with part of the broccoli and béchamel. Continue with the layers until all ingredients are used, ending with béchamel and a drizzle of EVO oil. Bake for 30 minutes.

Benefits: This dish is rich in vitamin C, antioxidants, and fiber thanks to the broccoli, while the oat milk béchamel provides a delicate supply of plant proteins. The vegetable margarine ensures a supply of "good" fats. A dish that reconciles taste and health, for a meal that does well for both body and soul.

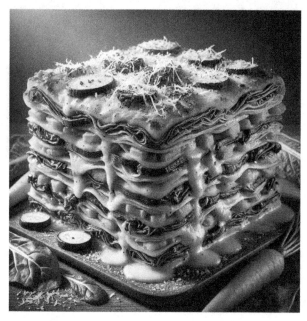

"Greenearth Lasagna: The Harmony of Escarole in a Vegetable Concert"

Ingredients for 4 people:

12 gluten-free lasagna sheets

2 heads of escarole

1 zucchini

1 carrot

2 onions

3 tablespoons of extra virgin olive oil

Salt and pepper to taste

500 ml of béchamel sauce (made with soy milk)

20 g of flour

20 g of margarine or olive oil

Salt to taste

Pepper to taste

Nutmeg to taste

100 g of grated vegan cheese

Procedure: Start by cleaning the escarole, zucchini, carrot, and onions, then chop them up and sauté in a pan with the oil. Season with salt and pepper and cook over medium heat for about 15 minutes until the vegetables are tender. For the béchamel: In a saucepan, heat the margarine or oil over medium heat.

When the margarine or oil is hot, add the flour, stirring constantly with a whisk to avoid lumps. This is your roux. Cook the roux for a couple of minutes, stirring constantly, to remove the taste of raw flour. Gradually start pouring in the soy milk, continuing to stir vigorously. Once all the milk is added, bring the sauce to a boil, continuing to stir. Lower the heat and simmer the béchamel until it thickens.

Add salt, pepper, and nutmeg to taste. Cook the béchamel for another 2-3 minutes, always stirring. At this point, your vegan béchamel is ready to use!

Remember that the consistency of the béchamel can be easily adjusted by adding more milk if you want a thinner sauce or cooking for longer if you prefer a thicker sauce.

In a baking dish, pour a drizzle of oil on the bottom, then lay the lasagna sheets, creating the first layer. Pour half of the vegetable sauté over the pasta, spreading well across the surface. Pour over a generous amount of béchamel and sprinkle with vegan cheese.

Repeat the operation creating another identical layer. Bake in a preheated oven at 180°C for 30 minutes, until the surface becomes golden and crispy.

Benefits: "Greenearth Lasagna" is an explosion of taste, thanks to the combination of escarole, zucchini, and carrot. Rich in vitamins A, C, K, and fiber from the vegetables used, it's a dish that nourishes and keeps the body healthy, thanks to the anti-inflammatory properties of the escarole. Additionally, the use of vegan cheese and lactose-free béchamel makes it suitable for those following a vegan diet or those who are lactose intolerant. A dish that is not only delicious but also good for you!

"Winter Aromatic Lasagna: A Meeting between Rice Béchamel and Porcini Mushrooms"

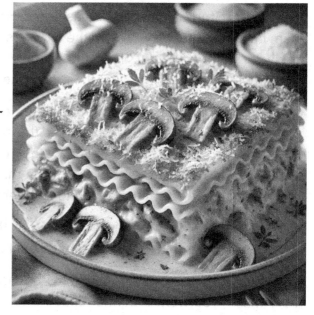

Ingredients for 4 people:

12 gluten-free lasagna sheets

500g of porcini mushrooms

1 onion

3 tablespoons of extra virgin olive oil

Salt and pepper to taste

500 ml of béchamel sauce (made with rice milk)

50 g of flour

50 g of vegetable margarine

Salt to taste

Nutmeg to taste

150 g of grated cheese for gratin

Procedure: Start by cleaning the porcini mushrooms carefully, then slice them thinly. Chop the onion and sauté it in a pan with the oil. Add the mushrooms, season with salt and pepper, and cook for about 20 minutes, or until the mushrooms are tender.

Meanwhile, prepare the béchamel sauce. In a saucepan, melt the margarine over medium heat.

As soon as the margarine is completely melted, add the flour, and mix well with a whisk to avoid lumps. Cook the flour and margarine together for a couple of minutes, stirring constantly: this will remove the raw flour taste.

At this point, start pouring in the rice milk slowly, continuing to stir to avoid lumps. Once all the milk is added, bring the béchamel to a boil. Keep stirring until it thickens. Now, season with salt and add a grating of nutmeg to flavor your béchamel. Continue cooking the béchamel for another 2-3 minutes, always stirring. At this point, your rice milk béchamel is ready to use!

Remember, if the béchamel is too thick, you can always add a bit more rice milk to reach the desired consistency. If you prefer it thicker, continue cooking for a few more minutes.

Preheat the oven to 180°C. Now, in a baking dish, create the first layer of lasagna. Pour over some of the sautéed mushrooms, then cover with a layer of béchamel. Repeat the process for all layers, until you finish the ingredients.

Finally, sprinkle the last layer with grated cheese. Bake for about 30 minutes, or until the lasagna is golden and well gratinated.

Benefits: The "Winter Aromatic Lasagna" is a reinterpretation of the classic Italian dish. Porcini mushrooms, rich in antioxidants and B vitamins, make this dish a real boon for the body. The béchamel sauce made with rice milk reduces the intake of saturated fats, making it a healthy choice. Finally, the final gratin in the oven gives this dish an unmistakable and irresistible taste.

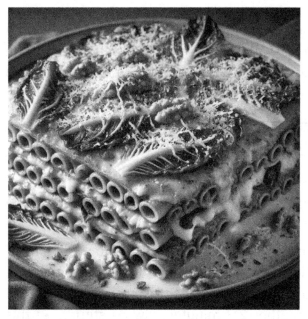

"Green Lasagna and Radicchio"

Ingredients for 4 people:

12 sheets of green lasagna

500g of radicchio

2 tablespoons of extra virgin olive oil

150g of chopped walnuts

150g of grated cheese for gratin

500 ml of béchamel sauce (made with rice milk)

50g of flour

50g of vegetable margarine

Salt and pepper to taste

Procedure: Start by cleaning the radicchio and cutting it into strips. In a pan, heat the oil and sauté the radicchio. After a few minutes, add the chopped walnuts and mix.

Prepare the béchamel sauce with rice milk: heat the rice milk with a knob of vegetable butter, add the flour, and stir until you get a thick cream. Season with salt and pepper.

Preheat the oven to 180°C. In a baking dish, create the first layer of green lasagna sheets. Pour over some of the sautéed radicchio and walnuts, then cover with the béchamel sauce. Repeat for all layers, finishing with the béchamel.

Finally, sprinkle the last layer with the grated cheese. Bake for about 30 minutes, or until the lasagna turns golden and gratinates.

Benefits: The "Green Lasagna and Radicchio" combines the slightly bitter taste of radicchio and the crunchiness of walnuts, balanced by the rice milk béchamel. Radicchio is a powerful anti-inflammatory, rich in vitamin K and antioxidants, while walnuts are a source of Omega-3. This dish offers an incredible combination of flavor and health.

"Restorative Soups"

"Chickpea and Rosemary Alchemic Soup: An Elixir of Health and Flavor"

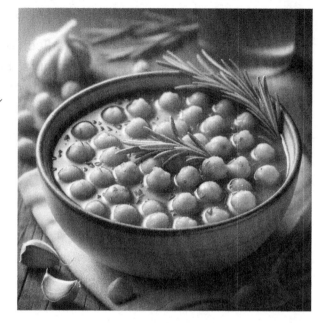

Ingredients for 4 people:

400g of dry chickpeas

1 tablespoon of extra virgin olive oil

2 cloves of garlic

1 sprig of rosemary

Salt and pepper to taste

1.5 liters of water

Procedure: Soak the chickpeas overnight. The next day, drain and set them aside. In a large pot, sauté the garlic in olive oil, add the chickpeas and rosemary, and sauté for a few minutes. Pour in the water, bring to a boil, lower the heat, and simmer for about 2 hours, or until the chickpeas are soft. Season with salt and pepper. Serve the soup hot.

Benefits: The "Chickpea and Rosemary Alchemic Soup" is a warm and nourishing dish, perfect for colder days. Chickpeas are an excellent source of plant proteins and fiber, while rosemary has potent anti-inflammatory properties. Together, they create a dish that not only warms the stomach but also supports the immune system and overall health.

This nutritious soup is a concentrate of vitamins and minerals, such as iron, which helps maintain cognitive functions, and vitamin K, which supports bone health. A true alchemy of health and flavor.

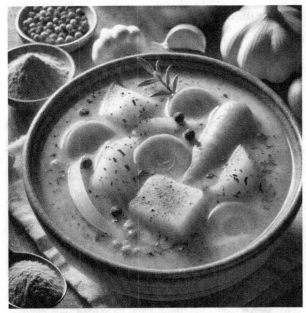

"Golden Health Soup: A Journey in Taste and Well-being"

Ingredients for 4 people:

3 medium potatoes

2 carrots

2 onions

2 cloves of garlic

1 tablespoon of turmeric

1 tablespoon of extra virgin olive oil

Salt and pepper to taste

1.5 liters of water

Procedure: Start by peeling and cubing the potatoes and carrots. Chop the onions and garlic. In a large pot, heat the oil and sauté the onion and garlic until they become translucent.

Add the potatoes and carrots to the pot, along with the turmeric, salt, and pepper. Mix well so that the spices blend with the vegetables. Cover with water and bring to a boil. Let it simmer for about 30 minutes or until the vegetables are tender.

Use an immersion blender to blend the soup into a creamy consistency. Taste and adjust for salt and pepper if necessary.

Benefits: The "Golden Health Soup" is an explosion of flavors and well-being. Potatoes and carrots, rich in vitamins A and C, contribute to strengthening the immune system. Turmeric, with its anti-inflammatory properties, is beneficial for the body, helping to prevent many chronic diseases. A delicious and healthy soup, perfect for indulging on cold winter days.

"Invigorating Farro and Spinach Soup: A Symphony of Nutrients"

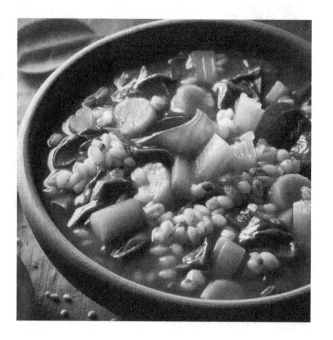

Ingredients for 4 people:

300g of farro

1 tablespoon of extra virgin olive oil

1 white onion, chopped

2 carrots, cubed

2 stalks of celery, cubed

150g of fresh spinach

1.5 liters of vegetable broth

Salt and pepper to taste

Procedure: Begin by soaking the farro for at least two hours. Meanwhile, in a large pot, heat the oil and add the onion, carrots, and celery. Sauté until the onion becomes transparent.

Rinse and drain the farro, then add it to the pot. Stir for a couple of minutes to lightly toast it. Pour in the vegetable broth, cover the pot, and cook over medium heat for about 30 minutes.

When the farro is almost cooked, add the washed and chopped spinach. Cook for another 10 minutes. Taste and adjust the seasoning with salt and pepper to your liking.

Benefits: The "Invigorating Farro and Spinach Soup" is a triumph of health and flavor. Farro is rich in fibers, proteins, and B vitamins, while spinach provides vitamins A, C, K, and iron. A rejuvenating and tasty meal.

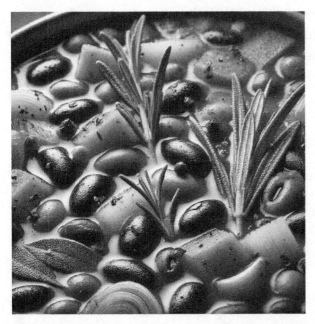

"Restorative Black Bean and Herb Soup: A Dive into Earthy Flavors"

Ingredients for 4 people:

400g of dried black beans

1 onion, chopped

2 cloves of garlic, chopped

2 carrots, cubed

2 stalks of celery, cubed

1 sprig of rosemary

1 sprig of sage

1.5 liters of water

Salt and pepper to taste

1 tablespoon of extra virgin olive oil

Procedure: Soak the black beans overnight. The next day, drain them and set aside. In a large pot, heat the oil and add the onion, garlic, carrots, and celery. Sauté until the onion becomes transparent.

Add the beans, rosemary, sage, water, salt, and pepper. Bring to a boil then reduce to a simmer. Cover the pot and let it cook for about two hours, stirring occasionally. If necessary, add more water.

Benefits: The "Restorative Black Bean and Herb Soup" is a celebration of flavors and health. Black beans are an excellent source of proteins, fibers, and B vitamins, while the aromatic herbs, in addition to providing an irresistible aroma, bring numerous benefits thanks to their antioxidant and anti-inflammatory properties. A great ally for your health, strengthening the immune system and aiding digestion.

"Cold Dishes: Rich and Complete Treasures"
"Quinoa, Farro, and Couscous: A Lively Taste"

"Delicious Quinoa Bowls: Chicken Strips, Pumpkin, and Cabbage in Aromatic Sauce"

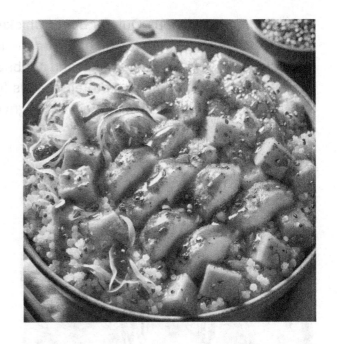

Ingredients for 4 people:

4 cups of quinoa

400g of chicken strips

1 medium pumpkin

1 cabbage

4 tablespoons of extra virgin olive oil

Soy sauce to taste

2 teaspoons of curry

Salt and pepper to taste

Procedure: Start by washing the quinoa under running water and then cook it in boiling salted water according to the package instructions.

Meanwhile, wash and cube the pumpkin, and slice the cabbage into thin strips. In a pan, heat a tablespoon of oil and cook the chicken strips until golden. Remove the chicken from the pan and add the pumpkin and cabbage, sautéing for about 10 minutes.

Drain the quinoa and transfer it to a large bowl, add the chicken, pumpkin, cabbage, soy sauce, curry, the rest of the oil, salt, and pepper. Mix well to combine all the ingredients.

Benefits: The "Delicious Quinoa Bowl: Chicken Strips, Pumpkin, and Cabbage in Aromatic Sauce" is an explosion of flavor and nutrition. The chicken provides high-quality proteins, while the pumpkin and cabbage bring vitamins and fibers. Quinoa, a superfood rich in fibers and proteins, adds further anti-inflammatory benefits to this nutritious and tasty dish. Perfect for a light dinner full of flavor and nutrients.

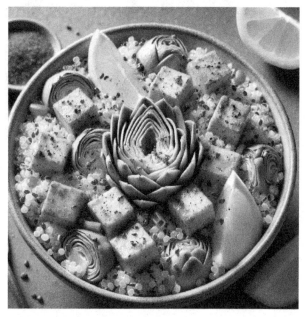

"Vibrant Quinoa Bowls with Artichokes and Tofu"

Ingredients for 4 people:

4 cups of quinoa

8 artichokes

400g of tofu

4 tablespoons of extra virgin olive oil

Juice of 2 lemons

2 teaspoons of sweet paprika

Salt and pepper to taste

Procedure: Start by washing the quinoa under running water and then cook it in boiling salted water according to the package instructions. Meanwhile, clean the artichokes by removing the hard leaves and the fuzzy center, then cut them into thin wedges.

In a pan, heat a tablespoon of oil and add the artichokes. Cook for about 10 minutes, until they become soft, add the tofu cut into cubes and continue cooking for another 5 minutes. Add paprika, salt, and pepper to taste.

Drain the quinoa and transfer it to a large bowl, add the artichokes and tofu, the lemon juice, and the rest of the oil. Mix well to combine all the ingredients.

Benefits: The "Vibrant Quinoa Bowl with Artichokes and Tofu" is a nutritious and flavorful recipe. Quinoa, artichokes, and tofu are rich in fibers and proteins, contributing to a balanced meal. Moreover, artichokes are known for their anti-inflammatory properties. A tasty and healthy option for a light lunch or dinner.

"Revival Bowls: Crunchy Farro & Fantasy with Goat Cheese and Parsley Sauce"

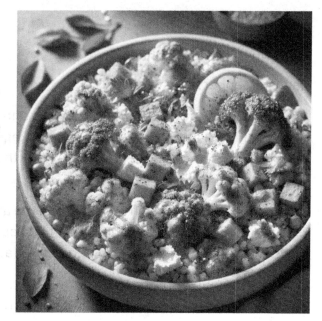

Ingredients for 4 people:

400g of farro

1 medium cauliflower

2 large, sweet potatoes

400g of goat cheese

Extra virgin olive oil, salt, and pepper to taste

1 bunch of fresh parsley

The juice of 1 lemon

Procedure: Cook the farro in plenty of salted water according to the package instructions. While the farro is cooking, cut the cauliflower into small florets and the sweet potatoes into cubes.

Heat some oil in a large pan and add the cauliflower and sweet potatoes. Sauté over medium-high heat until they become golden and crispy.

In the meantime, prepare the parsley sauce: wash and finely chop the parsley, then mix it with the lemon juice, a generous drizzle of olive oil, salt, and pepper.

Once the farro is ready, drain and let it cool. In a large bowl, mix the farro with the crispy cauliflower, sweet potatoes, and crumbled goat cheese. Finally, dress with the parsley sauce.

Benefits: This "Revival Bowl" is an explosion of flavors and nutrients. The farro provides proteins and fibers, while the cauliflower and sweet potatoes, sautéed to be crispy, offer vitamins, minerals, and an unmistakable taste. The goat cheese adds a touch of creaminess and a good dose of proteins. The parsley sauce brings a note of freshness and vitality, in addition to being rich in vitamin C. A lunch that stimulates the senses and nourishes the body, for a day full of energy.

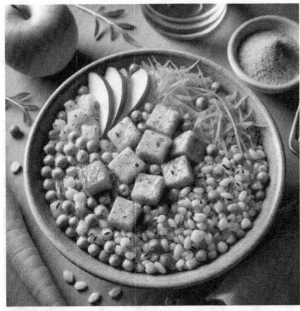

"Harmony Bowls: A World Tour in a Bowl of Farro"

Ingredients for 4 people:

400g of pearled farro

2 apples

400g of tofu

2 teaspoons of turmeric

4 carrots

400g of fresh peas

Extra virgin olive oil, salt, and pepper to taste

Procedure: Start by boiling the farro in salted water for about 20 minutes, or until it is al dente. Meanwhile, dice the tofu and apples, and grate the carrots.

Once cooked, drain the farro and rinse under cold water to stop the cooking process. In a large pan, heat a drizzle of olive oil and add the tofu, along with the turmeric, salt, and pepper. Sauté until the tofu turns golden.

In a large bowl, combine the farro, tofu, apples, grated carrots, and fresh peas. Mix well and taste, adding salt and pepper if necessary. Serve your farro bowls with a drizzle of raw olive oil.

Benefits: This "Harmony Bowl" represents a perfect balance of flavors and nutrition. Farro is a valuable source of fibers, proteins, and minerals, while tofu provides high-quality plant proteins. Apples and carrots contribute a supply of vitamins and antioxidants, while turmeric, with its anti-inflammatory properties, adds a touch of spice and health to the dish. This bowl is a true boon for the body and spirit!

"Mediterranean Bowl with Tuna: Couscous with Olive Fragrance and a Touch of the Sea"

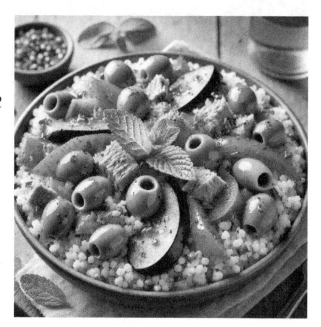

Ingredients for 4 people:

400g of couscous

2 eggplants

2 red bell peppers

200g of pitted green olives

2 onions

4 cloves of garlic

8 tablespoons of extra virgin olive oil (EVO)

300g of fresh tuna

Salt and pepper to taste

Fresh mint for garnish

Procedure: Start by preparing the couscous according to the package instructions.

Meanwhile, dice the eggplants, bell peppers, and tuna. Chop the onions and garlic and slice the olives into rounds.

In a large pan, sauté the onion in oil, then add the garlic. Add the vegetables, tuna, and olives, season with salt and pepper, cover, and cook for about 15 minutes, stirring occasionally.

When the vegetables and tuna are cooked, add the couscous to the pan and mix well to combine all the ingredients.

Benefits: The "Mediterranean Bowl with Tuna" offers a mix of anti-inflammatory ingredients such as olive oil, rich in monounsaturated fats, and olives, a source of vitamin E. Bell peppers, eggplants, and tuna provide fibers, proteins, and vitamins, contributing to the well-being of the digestive system and the maintenance of muscle mass. A bowl full of taste and health, taking your mind to the warm coasts of the Mediterranean, accompanied by the unique and unmistakable flavor of fresh tuna.

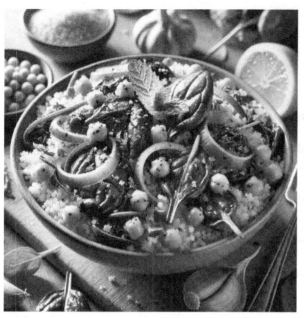

"Green Bowls: The Gentle Whisper of Couscous and Spinach"

Ingredients for 4 people:

400g of couscous

400g of fresh spinach

200g of precooked chickpeas

2 red onions

4 cloves of garlic

8 tablespoons of extra virgin olive oil (EVO)

Salt and pepper to taste

2 lemons

Fresh mint for garnish

Procedure: Follow the instructions on the package to prepare the couscous.

Meanwhile, clean and wash the spinach. Chop the onion and garlic and heat them in a pan with the EVO oil. Add the chickpeas and spinach, season with salt and pepper, and cook for about 10 minutes.

When the spinach is cooked, add the couscous to the pan and mix well to combine the ingredients. Finish with grated lemon zest and juice. Garnish with fresh mint leaves.

Benefits: A source of anti-inflammatory nutrients, thanks to the presence of spinach, rich in vitamin K, and chickpeas, an excellent source of plant proteins. A light, yet flavorful and nutritious dish that respects the delicate balance between well-being and taste.

"Cold Pasta: Summer is Coming"

"Farfalle in the Wind: A Sensory Journey through Whole Grains and Countryside Freshness"

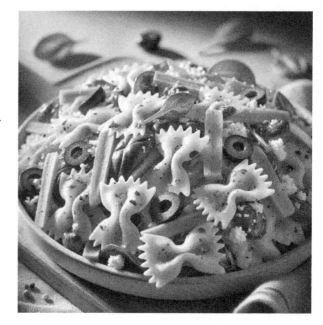

Ingredients for 4 people:

400g of wholemeal farfalle pasta

200g of fresh ricotta

4 medium carrots

200g of fresh baby spinach

100g of pitted black olives

Procedure: Begin our sensory journey by bringing a pot of salted water to a boil. Dive of wholemeal farfalle pasta into the boiling water, letting them dance for the time indicated on the package to ensure an al dente cooking.

Meanwhile, dedicate ourselves to preparing our countryside freshness: clean the carrots and reduce them to thin ribbons with the help of a vegetable peeler. Thoroughly wash the baby spinach and gently dry it. Finally, chop the black olives.

When the bow ties are ready, drain and cool them under a stream of cold water to stop the cooking. Place them in a large bowl and add the ricotta, carrot ribbons, baby spinach, and olives. Mix carefully to blend all the ingredients.

Refrigerate our pasta salad for at least one hour before serving. This will allow the flavors to meld perfectly, creating a fresh and tasty dish, perfect for the warmer days.

Benefits: This recipe is a true concentrate of anti-inflammatory nutrients. Whole wheat pasta is rich in fiber, which aids digestion and provides a sense of satiety. Ricotta is a source of low-fat proteins, while carrots, baby spinach, and olives are packed with vitamins and antioxidants. A delicious dish that nourishes both body and spirit.

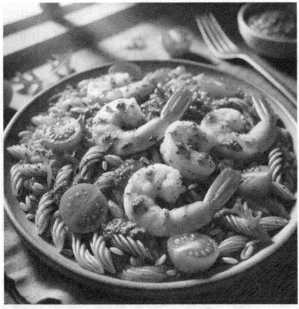

"Farro Dance: Marine Fusion of Pesto and Shellfish"

Ingredients for 4 people:

400g of farro pasta

For the Arugula Pesto:

100g of arugula

50g of pine nuts

Extra virgin olive oil

Salt

400g of shrimp

200g of cherry tomatoes

Procedure: First, bring a large pot of salted water to a boil and cook the farro pasta according to the package instructions.

Meanwhile, prepare our pesto. Wash the arugula and place it in a blender with the pine nuts, a pinch of salt, and enough olive oil to create a smooth and velvety cream.

Clean the shrimp by removing the shell and intestine. In a pan, heat a drizzle of olive oil and cook the shrimp for a couple of minutes on each side until they turn pink and tender. Remove the shrimp from the pan and set aside.

In the meantime, halve the cherry tomatoes and add them to the pan, cooking over medium heat until they start to soften.

Once the pasta is cooked, drain it and cool it under cold running water. Once cooled, mix the pasta with the arugula pesto, add the shrimp and cherry tomatoes, and gently mix.

Benefits: Farro is an excellent source of fiber and helps to keep the heart healthy. Arugula and cherry tomatoes are full of antioxidants, while pine nuts and shrimp provide high-quality proteins. A healthy and tasty recipe perfect for summer days.

"Fantastic Fusilli: The Symphony of Black Kale and Turmeric Tofu"

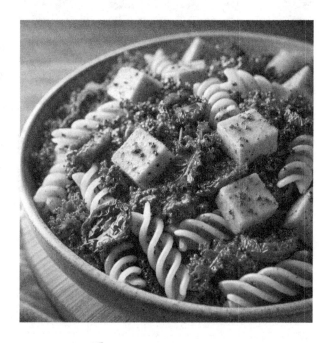

Ingredients for 4 people:

400g of gluten-free fusilli

200g of black kale

100g of sun-dried tomatoes

200g of tofu (or Feta, depending on your personal taste)

1 teaspoon of turmeric

Extra virgin olive oil

Salt and pepper

Procedure: Start by bringing a pot of water to a boil. When boiling, add a pinch of salt and the gluten-free fusilli. Cook the pasta according to the package instructions, then drain and cool it under cold water.

Meanwhile, wash the black kale, remove the ribs, and steam it until tender. Put the black kale in a blender, add a drizzle of olive oil, salt, and pepper to taste, and blend until you get a smooth pesto.

Cut the tofu into cubes and warm it in a non-stick pan with a drizzle of olive oil. When golden, add the turmeric and mix well to let the tofu absorb the flavors.

Rehydrate the sun-dried tomatoes in hot water for a few minutes, then cut them into pieces.

Finally, in a large bowl, combine the fusilli, black kale pesto, sun-dried tomatoes, and turmeric tofu. Mix well to blend all the ingredients.

Benefits: This recipe offers a rich mix of nutrients, thanks to the protein contribution of tofu, the anti-inflammatory properties of turmeric, and the vitamins A, C, K found in black kale. A dish that dances between the essence of the earth and the embrace of nature.

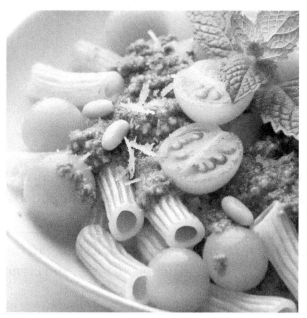

"Summer Cold Pasta: A Concert of Yellow Cherry Tomatoes and Mint Pesto"

Ingredients for 4 people:

400g of short pasta (e.g., penne rigate)

200g of yellow cherry tomatoes

A bunch of fresh mint

70g of pine nuts

1 clove of garlic

80g of Parmigiano Reggiano

100ml of extra virgin olive oil

Salt and pepper to taste

Procedure: Boil a pot of salted water and cook the pasta following the package instructions for al dente cooking. Meanwhile, wash and halve the yellow cherry tomatoes.

For the mint pesto, combine in a blender the mint, pine nuts, garlic, Parmigiano, oil, salt, and pepper. Blend until you get a smooth mixture.

Drain the pasta and rinse it under cold water to stop the cooking process. In a large bowl, combine the pasta, cherry tomatoes, and mint pesto, mixing well to blend all the ingredients. Let it rest in the fridge for at least an hour before serving.

Benefits: This dish is a true summer delight, fresh and light. Cold pasta is an excellent source of complex carbohydrates, which provide long-term energy. Yellow cherry tomatoes are rich in vitamin C and lycopene, a powerful antioxidant. The mint pesto, in addition to giving a refreshing flavor to the dish, contains pine nuts, a good source of monounsaturated and polyunsaturated fatty acids, beneficial for heart health. Finally, mint has digestive and antibacterial properties.

"Poke: From East to West"

"Japanese Poke: The Embrace of Brown Rice, Salmon, Mango, and Wakame Seaweed"

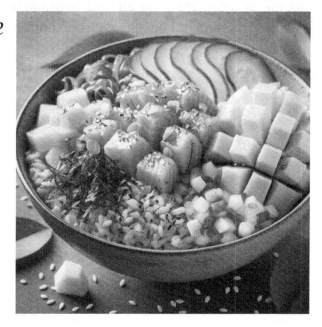

Ingredients for 4 people:

400g of whole grain brown rice

400g of fresh salmon fillet

2 ripe mangoes

2 cucumbers

50g of Wakame seaweed

2 tablespoons of sesame seeds

Soy sauce

Extra virgin olive oil

Juice of 1 lemon

Salt and pepper

Procedure: Start by cooking the whole grain brown rice according to the package instructions. Once cooked, let it cool completely.

Meanwhile, dice the salmon and place it in a bowl. Add the lemon juice, a drizzle of extra virgin olive oil, salt, and pepper, then mix well and let it marinate in the refrigerator for at least 30 minutes.

Peel the mangoes and cut them into cubes, then do the same with the cucumbers.

Rehydrate the Wakame seaweed in cold water for about 10 minutes, then drain and roughly chop it.

In a non-stick pan, lightly toast the sesame seeds.

Finally, to assemble the poke, start with a layer of whole grain brown rice, then add the salmon, mango, and cucumber cubes, the Wakame seaweed, and sprinkle with the toasted sesame seeds. Serve with a drizzle of soy sauce.

Benefits: This Japanese poke is a concentration of well-being: the proteins from the salmon, vitamins and antioxidants from the mango, fibers from the whole grain brown rice, and minerals from the Wakame seaweed come together in a delicious and nutritious dish, a real boon for our body.

"Eastern Elegance Poke: A Dance of Basmati Rice, Tuna, Edamame, Red Cabbage, and Toasted Almonds"

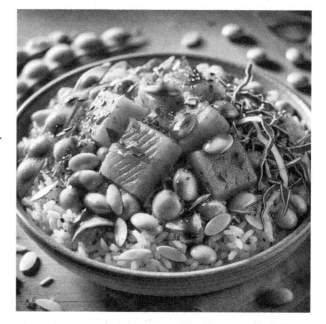

Ingredients for 4 people:

400g of Basmati rice

400g of fresh tuna

200g of edamame (green soybeans)

1 medium red cabbage

50g of almonds

Teriyaki sauce

Extra virgin olive oil

Juice of 1 lemon

Salt and pepper

Procedure: Cook the Basmati rice according to the package instructions, then let it cool.

Meanwhile, dice the tuna and place it in a bowl. Add the lemon juice, a drizzle of oil, salt, and pepper. Mix well and let it marinate in the refrigerator for at least 30 minutes.

Boil the edamame in salted water for about 5 minutes, then drain and let them cool.

Slice the red cabbage into thin strips. In a non-stick pan, toast the almonds until they are golden and crunchy.

To assemble the poke, distribute the Basmati rice into dishes, then add the marinated tuna, edamame, red cabbage, and sprinkle with the toasted almonds. Finish everything with a drizzle of Teriyaki sauce.

Benefits: This poke is a triumph of natural anti-inflammatories: the omega-3 from the tuna, fibers from the red cabbage and Basmati rice, proteins from the edamame, and healthy fats from the almonds, in a delicious embrace of flavors and nutrients for your body.

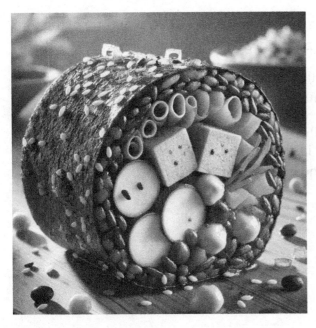

"Purple Passion Poke: A Dive into Black Rice, Tofu, Chickpeas, Zucchini, Carrots, and Nori Seaweed"

Ingredients for 4 people:

400g of black rice

300g of tofu

1 can of chickpeas

2 medium zucchinis

2 medium carrots

4 sheets of nori seaweed

Sesame sauce

Extra virgin olive oil

Juice of 1 lemon

Salt and pepper

Procedure: Start by cooking the black rice according to the package instructions, then let it cool.

Meanwhile, dice the tofu and place it in a bowl. Add the lemon juice, a drizzle of oil, salt, and pepper. Mix well and let it marinate in the refrigerator for at least 30 minutes.

Drain and rinse the chickpeas. Cut the zucchinis and carrots into thin sticks.

In a non-stick pan, cook the marinated tofu until golden, then set it aside.

Lay out the nori sheets and distribute a quarter of the black rice, a quarter of the tofu, a quarter of the chickpeas, and some zucchini and carrots on each.

Roll up the nori sheets with the filling inside and cut each roll in half. Finish everything with a drizzle of sesame sauce.

Benefits: A journey of taste and health, this poke bowl of black rice, tofu, chickpeas, zucchini, carrots, and nori seaweed is rich in antioxidants, proteins, and dietary fiber. A dish that delights the palate and nourishes the body.

Quote: *"The art of cooking is a form of love." - Jackie Kennedy.*

CHAPTER 11

"Original and Healthy Main Courses"

Diving into the world of "Original and Healthy Main Courses" immerses one in an ocean of intriguing options, perfect for experimenting and showcasing culinary skills. There's no more exhilarating moment than presenting a main course that defies tradition and steps beyond the boundaries of the ordinary.

The true magic of cooking unveils through the reinterpretation of classic dishes like baked fish, chicken, pan-seared turkey, and even seitan. These well-known and beloved ingredients offer a broad canvas for the chef's creativity to paint culinary surprises.

It's possible to reinvent fish with an exotic twist, discover an unexpected seasoning that revolutionizes chicken, present turkey in a tasty guise that defies expectations, or even transform seitan, often considered merely a meat substitute, into the undisputed protagonist of a main course.

And let's not forget about savory pies: the endless combinations of fillings offer a world of possibilities to astonish. Whether it's a classic filling or an unusual flavor pairing, the savory pie always represents a sophisticated and delicious option for a memorable main course.

In culinary arts, as in life, originality is the seasoning that distinguishes the common from the exceptional. At the grand feast of cooking, where every main course is a chapter of a tasty tale, every bite a surprise. And the only barrier is imagination.

"Baked Fish: A Journey to the Heart of the Sea"

"Golden Baked Cod: An Exotic Flavor Encounter"

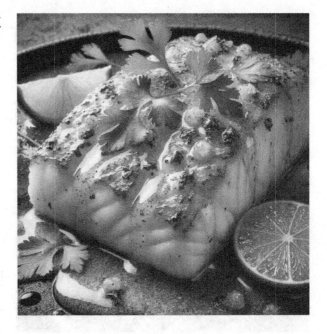

Ingredients for 4 servings:

4 cod fillets

1 lime

1 teaspoon of turmeric

2 tablespoons of extra virgin olive oil

2 tablespoons of acacia honey

Salt and pepper to taste

2 cloves of garlic

A bunch of fresh coriander

Procedure: Begin by preheating the oven to 180 degrees Celsius. Meanwhile, in a bowl, mix the lime juice, turmeric, honey, oil, chopped garlic, salt, and pepper to create an exotic marinade. Immerse the cod fillets in the marinade, making sure they are completely covered. Let them rest for 15-20 minutes to absorb all the flavors.

Place the cod fillets on a baking tray lined with parchment paper and bake for 12-15 minutes, or until the fish flakes easily with a fork. Garnish with fresh coriander before serving.

Benefits: This "Golden Baked Cod" combines the anti-inflammatory power of turmeric with the lightness of cod, an excellent source of proteins and omega-3. The addition of lime and coriander brings an exotic touch that will pleasantly surprise your palate.

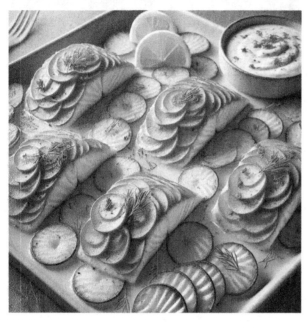

"Red Salmon Encrusted: A Dance of Flavors from the Deep Blue"

Ingredients for 4 servings:

4 salmon fillets

2 red potatoes

A bunch of dill

3 tablespoons of extra virgin olive oil

Salt and pepper to taste

2 lemons

200 ml of lactose-free cooking cream

Procedure: Preheat the oven to 180°C. While the oven heats up, wash and scrape the red potatoes. Slice them into very thin rounds, using a mandoline or a sharp knife.

Arrange the salmon fillets in a baking dish and season them with salt, pepper, and a drizzle of oil. Cover each fillet with potato slices, slightly overlapping them to create a 'scale' effect. Bake for 15-20 minutes, or until the potatoes are golden and crispy.

Meanwhile, prepare the sauce. In a saucepan, heat the cream over medium heat. Add chopped dill, the juice of one lemon, salt, and pepper. Simmer for 5-10 minutes, or until the sauce has slightly thickened. Once cooked, serve the salmon with the dill sauce and a slice of lemon.

Benefits: The "Red Salmon Encrusted" provides a rich supply of Omega-3s, natural anti-inflammatories, while the red potatoes offer an excellent dose of vitamin C and antioxidants. The dill sauce adds a fresh and aromatic touch that enhances the natural flavors of the fish. A true delight for the palate!

"Mediterranean Swordfish: A Dive into Mint, Eggplant, and Yellow Cherry Tomatoes"

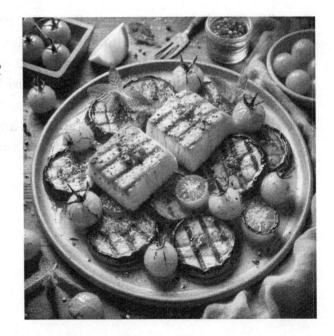

Ingredients for 4 servings:

4 swordfish fillets

2 medium eggplants

200g yellow cherry tomatoes

A bunch of fresh mint

4 tablespoons of extra virgin olive oil

Salt and pepper to taste

Juice of 1 lemon

Procedure: Start by preheating the oven to 200°C. While the oven heats up, slice the eggplants into thin slices and the cherry tomatoes in half. Arrange the eggplants and tomatoes in a baking dish, season with half the oil, salt, and pepper, and bake for 15-20 minutes, or until the eggplants are tender and golden.

Meanwhile, season the swordfish fillets with the remaining oil, lemon juice, salt, pepper, and half of the chopped mint. Heat a non-stick pan and cook the swordfish for 3-4 minutes on each side, or until it is nicely browned and cooked through.

Serve the swordfish fillets on a bed of roasted eggplants and cherry tomatoes, garnished with the remaining chopped fresh mint.

Benefits: This dish is a true explosion of flavors and nutritional benefits. Swordfish is an excellent source of high biological value proteins, B vitamins, and minerals such as selenium. Eggplants provide a good amount of fiber, which aids digestion and cholesterol control, and are rich in antioxidants. Yellow cherry tomatoes are an excellent source of vitamin C and lycopene, a powerful antioxidant. Finally, mint adds a touch of freshness and has digestive and antioxidant properties. A dish that combines well-being and taste, perfect for a summer dinner.

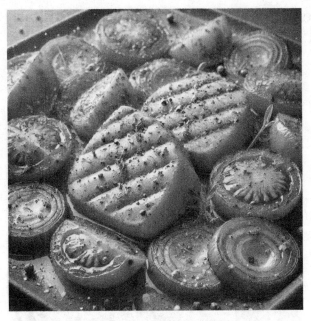

"Mediterranean Aromatic Tuna: A Flavor Explosion from the Heart of the Sea"

Ingredients for 4 servings:

4 fresh tuna steaks

2 ripe tomatoes

1 red onion

2 tablespoons of extra virgin olive oil

Salt and pepper to taste

1 lemon

2 teaspoons of dried oregano

Procedure: Preheat the oven to 200°C. Meanwhile, wash and slice the tomatoes, and chop the red onion.

Place the tuna steaks in a baking dish and sprinkle them with oregano, salt, and pepper. Arrange the tomatoes and onion over and around the fish. Season with olive oil and lemon juice.

Bake for about 15-20 minutes, or until the tuna is cooked to your liking. Remember that the cooking time may vary depending on the thickness of the tuna steaks.

Benefits: This recipe offers a riot of flavors typical of the Mediterranean diet. Oregano, with its anti-inflammatory properties, perfectly complements the freshness of the tuna, a fish rich in Omega-3. Lemon adds a touch of acidity that balances the entire preparation, offering a healthy, nutritious, and incredibly tasty dish.

"Aromatic Baked Sea Bream with Pumpkin and Zucchini: An Explosion of Flavors from Sea to Land"

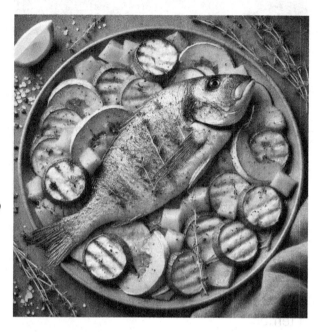

Ingredients for 4 servings:

4 fresh, cleaned, and scaled sea breams

1 small pumpkin

2 zucchinis

2 tablespoons of extra virgin olive oil

1 bunch of fresh thyme

Salt and pepper to taste

1 lemon

Procedure: Preheat the oven to 200°C. Meanwhile, clean and slice the pumpkin and zucchinis thinly.

Line a baking dish with parchment paper and arrange a layer of the vegetables on the bottom. Season with salt, pepper, and a tablespoon of oil. Place the sea breams on top, add the remaining thyme, salt, pepper, and the rest of the oil. Finish with the remaining vegetables and a drizzle of lemon juice.

Bake in the oven for about 30-35 minutes, or until the sea bream is well cooked and the vegetables are tender.

Benefits: "Pleasures from Sea to Garden" is a symphony of flavors and nutrients. Sea bream, with its Omega-3 content, is a great ally for heart health. The vegetables, rich in vitamins and antioxidants, complete the dish making it a celebration of well-being. Thyme, with its anti-inflammatory properties, adds a unique aromatic touch, wrapping everything in a delicious harmony of tastes. Rich in Omega-3, vitamins, and antioxidants, this dish is a true feast for the senses and a boon for health!

"Chicken and Turkey: Slow Heat Cooking"

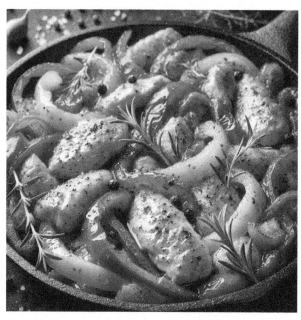

"Herb-Scented Chicken and Turkey Sauté: An Explosion of Flavor and Health"

Ingredients for 4 servings:

1 kg of chicken, cut into pieces

2 red bell peppers

2 yellow bell peppers

3 tablespoons of extra virgin olive oil

1 sprig of rosemary

1 sprig of thyme

Salt and pepper to taste

Procedure: Start by cleaning and slicing the bell peppers into strips. Heat a large pan and pour in the olive oil. Once the oil is hot, add the chicken and turkey pieces, browning them on all sides. Then, add the peppers and the bouquet of aromatic herbs, season with salt and pepper.

Cook over medium heat for about 30 minutes, stirring occasionally, add a couple of tablespoons of water if needed. When the chicken and turkey are nicely browned and the peppers are soft, your dish is ready. Serve hot, accompanied by a fresh salad.

Benefits: A dish full of flavor, but also benefits for health. Chicken and turkey are rich in lean proteins, while the bell peppers are an important source of vitamin C, perfect for a healthy and balanced diet. Furthermore, the aromatic herbs provide flavor without adding fats or calories. A delicious and healthy dish, great for a lunch or family dinner.

"Citrus and Thyme Chicken Bites: A Vitamin-Rich and Fresh Cocktail"

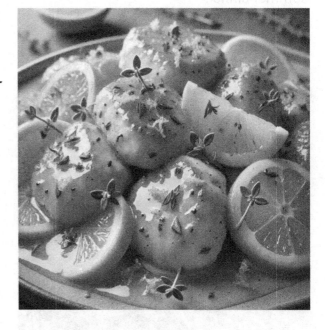

Ingredients for 4 servings:

1 kg of chicken breast

2 oranges

2 lemons

1 bunch of fresh thyme

3 tablespoons of extra virgin olive oil

Salt and pepper to taste

Procedure: Start by cutting the chicken breast into equally sized bites. Season with salt and pepper. Heat a pan with olive oil and, once hot, add the chicken bites, browning them on all sides.

Meanwhile, wash and dry the oranges and lemons. Grate the zest of one orange and one lemon and squeeze the juice of all the oranges and lemons. Add the zest and juices to the pan with the chicken, along with half of the chopped thyme bunch.

Lower the heat and cook for another 10-15 minutes, or until the chicken is cooked through and the sauce has slightly thickened. Just before serving, sprinkle the chicken bites with the remaining chopped thyme.

Benefits: This dish is an explosion of flavors and vitamins. Chicken provides high-quality proteins, essential for maintaining muscle mass. The citrus fruits, in addition to giving a touch of freshness and lightness to the dish, are rich in vitamin C, a powerful antioxidant. Thyme, in addition to giving a unique aroma to the dish, has antibacterial properties. A light, tasty, and nutritious dish, perfect for a lunch or summer dinner.

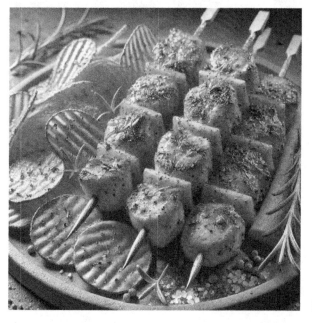

"Eastern Chicken in Overnight Marinade and Aromatic Sweet Potato Chips: A Flavor Journey from East to West"

Ingredients for 4 servings:

For the skewers:

1 kg of chicken breast

600g of natural yogurt

3 teaspoons of turmeric

3 teaspoons of sweet paprika

2 teaspoons of cumin

Salt to taste

For the sweet potato chips:

4 large, sweet potatoes

2 tablespoons of extra virgin olive oil

1 teaspoon of chopped rosemary

Salt to taste

Procedure: Start by preparing the chicken marinade: mix the yogurt with the spices and salt in a large bowl. Add the diced chicken breast and let it marinate in the refrigerator overnight.

The next day, thread the chicken onto skewers and bake in a preheated oven at 200°C (392°F) for about 20 minutes, until the chicken is golden and crispy.

For the sweet potato chips, start by cleaning and slicing the potatoes thinly. Place them in a bowl and season with oil, chopped rosemary, and salt. Arrange the slices on a baking sheet lined with parchment paper, without overlapping, and bake in the oven at 200°C (392°F) for about 20 minutes, or until crispy. Serve the dish hot and get ready for a burst of flavor.

Benefits: A dish full of exotic flavors and health benefits. This dish is a boon for health: chicken provides high-quality proteins, spices like turmeric and cumin have anti-inflammatory properties, and yogurt is rich in probiotics. Sweet potatoes, meanwhile, are a source of vitamins A and C, and are rich in fiber. A taste journey between the East and West, taking care of our well-being.

"Turkey in the Art of Spring: A Dance of Flavor and Health"

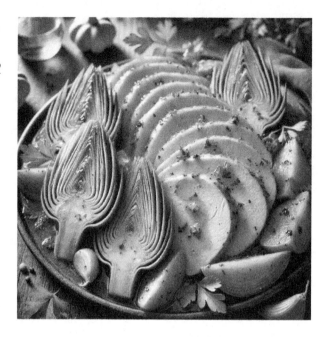

Ingredients for 4 servings:

800g of turkey slices

8 fresh artichokes

3 tablespoons of extra virgin olive oil

2 cloves of garlic

Juice of 1 lemon

Salt and pepper to taste

Fresh parsley to taste

Procedure: Clean the artichokes by removing the tougher outer leaves and cutting them into wedges. Keep them in water with lemon juice to prevent them from blackening.

In a large pan, heat the oil and garlic. When the garlic is golden, add the drained artichokes and sauté for a few minutes. Add a little water, cover the pan, and cook over medium heat for about 15 minutes.

Meanwhile, lightly beat the turkey slices to make them thinner, then add them to the pan with the artichokes. Season with salt and pepper and cook for another 10 minutes, turning frequently.

Finish with a sprinkling of chopped parsley and serve your "Turkey in the Art of Spring" hot.

Benefits: The combination of turkey and artichokes in this recipe offers a perfect balance of lean proteins and fiber, making this dish not only tasty but also beneficial for health. Artichokes are known for their antioxidant and purifying properties, while turkey is an excellent source of B vitamins.

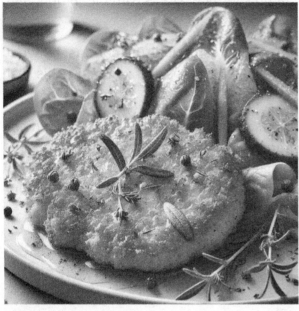

"Oven-Baked Golden Turkey Cutlets with Spring Salad"

Ingredients for 4 servings:

For the cutlets:

800g of turkey slices

2 or 3 eggs (depending on size)

200g of breadcrumbs

Aromatic herbs (rosemary, thyme, sage) to taste

Salt and pepper to taste

For the salad:

200g of lamb's lettuce or salad of your choice

1 carrot

1 cucumber

Extra virgin olive oil, lemon, salt, and pepper for dressing

Procedure: Prepare the turkey cutlets by lightly beating them and then dipping them into the beaten egg. Mix the breadcrumbs with the chopped aromatic herbs, salt, and pepper and use this mixture to bread both sides of the turkey slices.

Arrange the cutlets on a baking tray lined with parchment paper and bake at 200°C (392°F) for about 15 minutes, or until they are golden and crispy.

Meanwhile, wash and dry the lamb's lettuce, carrot, and cucumber. Julienne the carrot and cucumber and mix with the lamb's lettuce. Dress with oil, lemon, salt, and pepper to taste.

Serve the hot turkey cutlets accompanied by the fresh salad. The contrast between the crunchiness of the turkey and the freshness of the salad will make this dish irresistible.

Benefits: Oven-Baked Golden Turkey Cutlets with Spring Salad are a balanced and nutritious option, rich in lean proteins, vitamins, and minerals. Turkey provides high-quality protein and B vitamins, while raw vegetables contribute fiber and vitamins. A dish that combines taste and well-being, perfect for those looking for healthy cuisine without sacrificing flavor.

"Jumping Turkey Meatballs: A Dive into the Mediterranean with Tomato Sauce and Herbs"

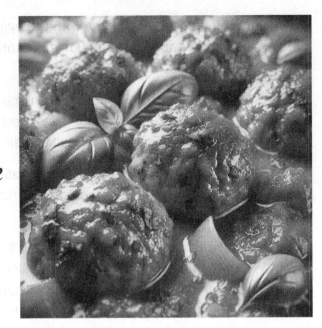

Ingredients for 4 servings:

For the meatballs:

1 kg of ground turkey

1 or 2 eggs (depending on size)

100g of breadcrumbs

4 tablespoons of grated Parmesan cheese

Salt and pepper to taste

Fresh parsley to taste

For the sauce:

1 can of peeled tomatoes

1 onion

2 cloves of garlic

Extra virgin olive oil to taste

Salt and pepper to taste

Fresh basil to taste

Procedure: Mix the ground turkey with the egg, breadcrumbs, Parmesan, chopped parsley, salt, and pepper. Work the mixture until you have a uniform dough and then form small meatballs.

For the sauce, sauté the chopped onion and garlic in a bit of olive oil in a large skillet. Add the peeled tomatoes and cook over medium heat for 15-20 minutes. Season with salt and pepper and add torn basil leaves.

In a skillet with a bit of oil, brown the meatballs on all sides. Once they are nicely golden, add the tomato sauce and let cook for another 10-15 minutes, or until the meatballs are fully cooked.

Benefits: This dish is a high-quality protein source thanks to the turkey, while the tomato sauce provides vitamin C and lycopene, a powerful antioxidant. The breadcrumbs and Parmesan add flavor without weighing down the dish, making it perfect for a light yet nutritious dinner. Additionally, basil and parsley not only add freshness and aroma but also have antibacterial and anti-inflammatory properties.

"Savory Pies: Balance and Pleasure of the Palate"

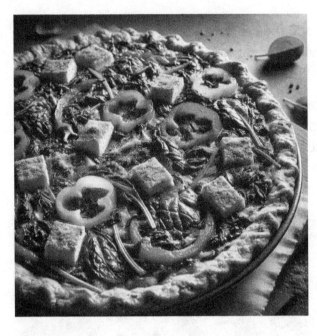

"Savory Pie: The Anti-Inflammatory Rainbow"

For this recipe, a pie dish with a diameter of about 23-26 cm is ideal.

For the crust:

200g of oat flour

100g of extra virgin olive oil

50ml of water

A pinch of salt

For the filling:

200g of fresh spinach

1 red bell pepper

1 yellow bell pepper

1 tablespoon of turmeric

2 eggs

200g of tofu

Procedure: Start by preparing the crust. In a bowl, combine the oat flour, olive oil, water, and salt. Work the dough until smooth, then spread it in a pie dish lined with parchment paper.

For the filling, cook the spinach in a pan with a bit of oil until wilted. Cut the bell peppers into strips and add them to the spinach, cooking for another 5 minutes. Add the turmeric and mix well.

In a separate bowl, beat the eggs and add the crumbled tofu. Combine the spinach and bell pepper mixture and stir everything together. Pour the filling onto the crust and bake at 180°C for 25-30 minutes or until the pie is golden.

Benefits: This pie is a true treasure trove of nutrients. Rich in proteins from tofu and eggs, vitamin C from bell peppers, and antioxidants from turmeric and spinach. It's a balanced, tasty dish that helps reduce inflammation.

"Savory Pie: An Anti-inflammatory Explosion of Broccoli and Salmon"

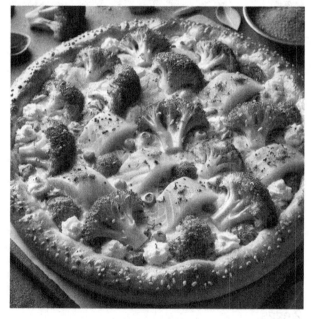

For this recipe, it's ideal to use a pie dish with a diameter of about 24cm.

For the crust:

250g of whole wheat flour

125g of cold butter (lactose-free)

1 egg

A pinch of salt

For the filling:

250g of broccoli

200g of salmon fillet

1 tablespoon of turmeric

2 eggs

200g of ricotta

Procedure: Start by preparing the crust. In a bowl, mix the whole wheat flour, the cold cubed butter, the egg, and salt. Work the dough until it's homogeneous, then roll it out in a pie dish lined with baking paper.

For the filling, boil the broccoli in salted boiling water for 10 minutes, then drain and let it cool. Meanwhile, cook the salmon in a non-stick pan, then shred it.

In a separate bowl, beat the eggs and add the ricotta. Combine the broccoli, shredded salmon, and turmeric; mix until you have a homogeneous mixture. Pour the filling over the crust and bake at 180°C for about 30 minutes, or until golden.

Benefits: Our savory pie offers a winning combination of anti-inflammatory ingredients: salmon rich in omega-3, broccoli full of antioxidants, and turmeric with its healing properties. A dish that delights the palate and also promotes body health!

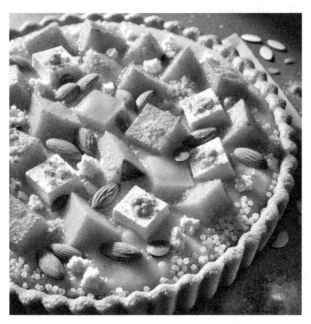

"Savory Pie: An Anti-inflammatory Delight of Pumpkin and Quinoa"

For this recipe, it's ideal to use a pie dish with a diameter of about 24cm.

For the crust:

200g of cooked quinoa

100g of ground almonds

2 eggs

A pinch of salt

For the filling:

500g of pumpkin

2 tablespoons of extra virgin olive oil

1 tablespoon of turmeric

200g of feta cheese

Procedure: For the crust, in a bowl mix the cooked quinoa, ground almonds, eggs, and salt. Work the dough until well combined and spread it in a 24cm pie dish.

For the filling, cut the pumpkin into cubes and cook in a pan with extra virgin olive oil and turmeric until soft. Let it cool.

In a separate bowl, crumble the feta cheese. Add the cooled pumpkin and mix well. Pour the filling over the quinoa base and bake at 180°C for about 30 minutes or until golden.

Benefits: This pie is a treasure trove of anti-inflammatory ingredients: quinoa, rich in protein and fiber; pumpkin, a source of vitamins and antioxidants; and turmeric, known for its anti-inflammatory properties. A delicious dish that nourishes both body and soul!

"Stuffed Bundles: A Triumph of Escarole, Raisins, Tofu, and Black Olives"

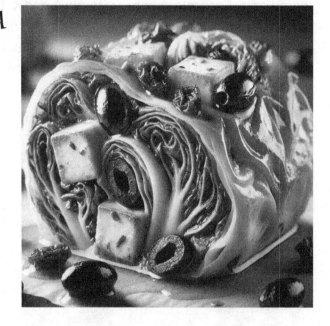

Ingredients for 4 people:

400g curly escarole

200g tofu

100g pitted black olives

50g raisins

2 cloves of garlic

Extra virgin olive oil as needed

Salt and pepper to taste

8 sheets of phyllo dough

Procedure: Start by soaking the raisins in warm water for about 10 minutes. Meanwhile, wash and clean the escarole, then cut it into strips. In a large pan, sauté the garlic in some oil, then add the escarole, chopped black olives, crumbled tofu, drained raisins, and a pinch of salt and pepper. Cook everything over medium heat for about 15 minutes, then let cool.

Lay out the phyllo dough sheets and place a portion of the escarole filling in the center of each. Fold the edges of the phyllo dough over themselves, forming the bundles. Bake at 180°C for about 15-20 minutes, or until golden.

Benefits: This dish offers a variety of nutrients thanks to its combination of ingredients. Escarole is rich in vitamin A and K, fiber, and antioxidants. The tofu, high in protein, adds a touch of sweetness to the dish, while the black olives and raisins provide a rich and deep flavor. Finally, extra virgin olive oil provides healthy monounsaturated fats. A balanced and healthy meal that is also tasty and satisfying!

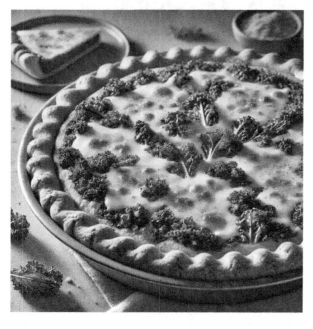

"Savory Pie: An Anti-Inflammatory Enchantment of Kale and Rice Flour"

For this recipe, it is ideal to use a pie dish with a diameter of about 24cm.

For the crust:

200g rice flour

100g water

50g extra virgin olive oil

A pinch of salt

For the filling:

200g kale

2 tablespoons extra virgin olive oil

1 teaspoon turmeric

200g lactose-free mozzarella

Procedure: For the crust, mix the rice flour, water, extra virgin olive oil, and salt in a bowl until you have a smooth and compact dough. Spread the dough into a 24cm diameter pie dish.

For the filling, cook the kale in a pan with extra virgin olive oil and turmeric until wilted. Let cool.

Dice the lactose-free mozzarella and combine it with the cooled kale in a separate bowl. Pour the filling over the rice flour base and bake at 180°C for about 30 minutes or until golden.

Benefits: This pie offers a powerful mix of anti-inflammatory ingredients: rice flour, rich in fiber; kale, a source of vitamins and minerals; and turmeric, with its anti-inflammatory properties. A delicious dish that satisfies and deeply nourishes!

"Seitan with Love and Flavor"

"Seitan in Flight: Revolutionary Scaloppine"

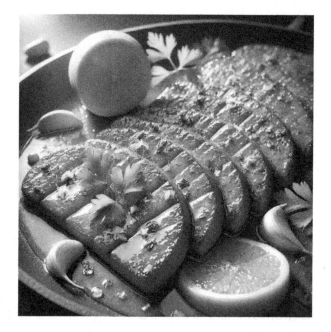

Ingredients for 4 servings:

400g seitan

2 cloves of garlic

Juice and zest of 1 organic lemon

2 tablespoons of extra virgin olive oil

Salt and pepper to taste

Fresh parsley

Procedure: Slice the seitan into half-centimeter thick slices. Heat the oil in a non-stick pan, add the crushed garlic and let it lightly brown. Place the seitan slices in the pan, cook for 3 minutes per side, then season with salt and pepper.

Grate the lemon zest and squeeze out the juice. When the seitan scaloppine are golden, add the lemon juice and grated zest, mixing well to flavor them. Finally, turn off the heat and sprinkle the scaloppine with chopped fresh parsley.

Benefits: The "Revolutionary Scaloppine" of seitan are a dish rich in plant-based proteins, a great alternative to meat. Seitan is known for its ability to reduce inflammation and improve heart health. Lemon, rich in vitamin C, and garlic, known for its anti-inflammatory properties, make this dish a concentration of health.

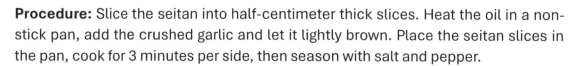

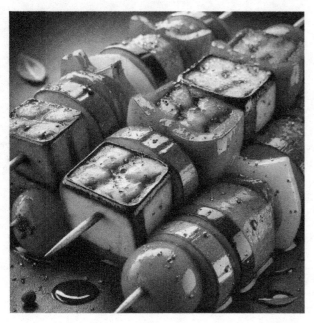

"Rainbow Seitan: Skewers of Seitan and Colorful Vegetables"

Ingredients for 4 servings:

400g seitan

2 colored bell peppers (1 red and 1 yellow)

1 eggplant

1 zucchini

2 tablespoons of extra virgin olive oil

Soy sauce

Salt and pepper to taste

Procedure: Cut the seitan and vegetables into approximately 2 cm cubes. Prepare the skewers by alternating seitan, bell peppers, eggplant, and zucchini. Season with a drizzle of oil and a bit of soy sauce; then, cook the skewers on a hot grill for 5-7 minutes per side, until well browned.

Finally, adjust with salt and pepper, and serve hot, perhaps accompanied by a fresh salad or brown rice.

Benefits: The "Rainbow Skewers" of seitan and vegetables are an extremely nutritious dish, rich in plant proteins, vitamins, and minerals. Seitan, in particular, is known for its anti-inflammatory properties and as an excellent source of protein. The colorful vegetables provide a variety of health-beneficial antioxidants, contributing to a balanced and tasty dish.

"Oriental Sensation Seitan: Seitan Bites with Creamy Asian Sauce"

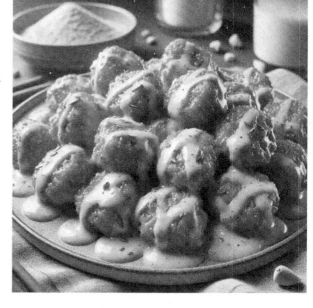

Ingredients for 4 servings:

400g seitan

2 tablespoons sesame oil

For the sauce:

200 ml coconut milk

2 tablespoons soy sauce

1 tablespoon green curry paste

1 teaspoon brown sugar

Procedure: Start by cutting the seitan into evenly sized bites. Heat the sesame oil in a pan and add the seitan, browning it until golden. Meanwhile, prepare the sauce: in a small pot, combine coconut milk, soy sauce, green curry paste, and brown sugar. Bring to a boil and let simmer for 5-10 minutes until it thickens.

Finally, pour the sauce over the seitan bites and stir well to ensure they are well coated. Serve hot, with a side of basmati rice or steamed vegetables.

Benefits: The "Seitan Bites with Creamy Asian Sauce" offer a valid alternative to animal proteins. Seitan is a source of plant proteins, while the creamy Asian sauce, thanks to coconut milk and green curry paste, introduces antioxidants and healthy fats. A delicious and nutritious dish that blends the oriental and western culinary traditions.

Quote: *"The food is the universal language of love." - Anthony Bourdain.*

CHAPTER 12

"Street Food at Your Home"

Welcome to a new chapter titled "Street Food at Your Home," designed to awaken the charm of an extraordinarily vibrant and diverse world of flavors. A virtual journey through the world's aromas, taking us on an exploration and reinterpretation of the lively universe of street food, all from the comfort of our kitchen.

Juicy burgers, from the classic meat version to revolutionary vegan dishes, or embracing wraps filled with fresh and colorful ingredients, or even the versatile sandwiches that can encompass flavors from land to sea. There's truly a world of possibilities waiting for you.

Imagine savoring the excitement of a street food stall in the tranquility of your home. Smelling the aroma that spreads as you prepare the perfect burger, the thrill of creating a wrap that encapsulates the best of Mediterranean flavors, or the satisfaction of biting into a vegetarian sandwich that explodes with taste.

This is the spirit of street food - simplicity, authenticity, the desire to share, and a passion for good food. But now, with a touch of 'home', an accent of familiarity and comfort, you can bring this experience into your own kitchen, creating and enjoying your favorite dishes in a homey setting. And don't forget, personalizing these dishes is a breeze: you can express your culinary personality and amaze your loved ones with your incredible creations.

Rediscover the pleasure of street food, without leaving your home. Remember, the culinary adventure is always at hand, and you never know where your next one will take you!

"Juicy and Good Burgers"

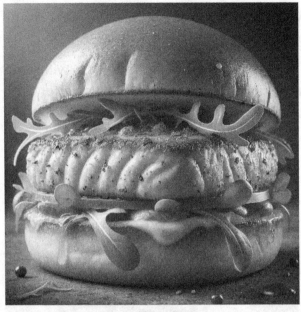

"Salmon Burger: An Explosion of Flavor from the Sea to Your Plate"

For 8 burgers:

800g of fresh salmon fillet

2 teaspoons of turmeric

4 tablespoons of extra virgin olive oil

Salt and pepper to taste

8 hamburger buns

Mixed salad greens (arugula, lettuce, etc.)

4 tablespoons of extra virgin olive oil

Juice of 1 lemon

Salt and pepper to taste

A teaspoon of light mayonnaise (optional)

Procedure: Start by cleaning the salmon fillet, removing the skin and bones. Then, cut it into cubes and transfer it to a mixer. Add turmeric, salt, pepper, and a tablespoon of oil. Blend everything until you get a homogeneous mixture.

Form 8 burgers and cook them in a non-stick pan with three tablespoons of olive oil. Cook for about 4 minutes per side, until they become golden.

Meanwhile, prepare the side salad: in a bowl, mix the greens with oil, lemon juice, salt, and pepper.

Serve the salmon burgers in the buns, with a bit of salad on the side. Enjoy the aroma of the sea and the refined taste of salmon combined with turmeric.

Benefits: Salmon is a rich source of omega-3, an essential fatty acid with anti-inflammatory properties. Combined with turmeric, known for its powerful anti-inflammatory and antioxidant effects, this salmon burger offers an explosion of health and flavor in every bite.

"Cod Burger with Grilled Zucchini on Whole Wheat Bread"

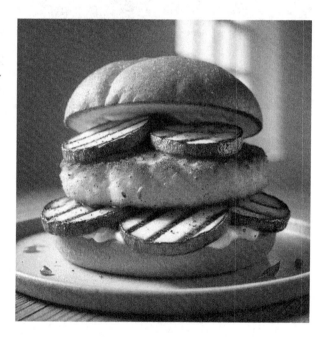

For 8 burgers:

800g of fresh cod

8 whole wheat hamburger buns

2 zucchinis

A bunch of fresh thyme

Salt and pepper

Extra virgin olive oil

1 egg

100g of breadcrumbs

A teaspoon of yogurt sauce (optional)

Procedure: Start by removing the flesh of the cod, being careful to remove all bones. Put the fish in a mixer with a pinch of salt, pepper, a tablespoon of oil, and the fresh thyme. Blend everything until you get a homogeneous mixture.

Transfer the mixture to a bowl, add the egg and breadcrumbs, and mix until combined. Form 8 burgers with your hands and place them on a tray. Let them rest in the fridge for at least 30 minutes.

Meanwhile, slice the zucchinis lengthwise and grill them on a hot griddle on both sides.

Heat a non-stick pan with a drizzle of oil. Cook the cod burgers for about 3-4 minutes per side or until they become golden. Toast the whole wheat buns in the same pan.

Assemble the burger by placing some grilled zucchini on the bottom of the bun, then the cod burger, and top with the other half of the bun.

Benefits: The choice of ingredients is key to this dish's benefits. Cod is a source of lean proteins, while whole wheat bread is rich in fiber. Grilled zucchinis add a touch of freshness and an additional supply of fiber and vitamins.

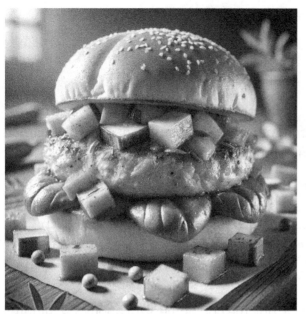

"Citrus-Flavored Chicken Burger with Sautéed Vegetables"

For 8 burgers:

800g of chicken breast

Grated zest of 1 orange and 1 lemon

8 hamburger buns

Salt and pepper

Extra virgin olive oil

1 egg

100g of breadcrumbs

For the side:

4 carrots

1 small-sized pumpkin

2 tablespoons of extra virgin olive oil

Salt and pepper

Procedure: For the burgers, grind the chicken breast in a mixer until finely minced. Transfer it to a bowl and add the grated zest of orange and lemon, salt, pepper, the egg, and breadcrumbs. Mix the ingredients well and form 8 burgers. Put them in the fridge to rest for at least 30 minutes.

Meanwhile, prepare the side. Clean and dice the carrots and pumpkin. Heat the oil in a pan and add the vegetables. Cook over medium heat for about 15-20 minutes, stirring occasionally, until the vegetables are cooked but still crunchy. Season with salt and pepper.

Heat a non-stick pan with a drizzle of oil and cook the chicken burgers for about 4-5 minutes per side, until they are well browned. Toast the buns on the same pan.

Serve the chicken burgers in the buns and accompany with vegetables.

Benefits: The citrus-flavored chicken burgers are a source of lean protein, and the vegetables provide high content of vitamins A and C, useful for the immune system and skin health.

"Herb-Infused Turkey Burgers with Grilled Cherry Tomatoes"

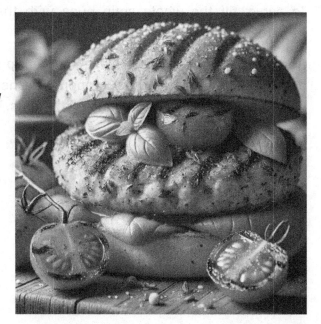

For 8 burgers:

800g of turkey breast

A handful of basil and mint leaves

8 whole grain hamburger buns

Salt and pepper

1 egg

100g of breadcrumbs

For the grilled cherry tomatoes:

16 cherry tomatoes

Extra virgin olive oil

Salt

Procedure: Start by grinding the turkey breast in a mixer until finely minced. Add basil and mint, salt, pepper, the egg, and breadcrumbs. Mix well and form 8 burgers. Put them in the fridge to rest for 30 minutes.

Meanwhile, prepare the cherry tomatoes. Cut them in half, season with oil and salt, and place them on a baking tray. Grill in a preheated oven at 200°C for 15-20 minutes or until golden.

Heat a non-stick pan with a drizzle of oil. Cook the burgers for 4-5 minutes per side, until golden. Toast the buns on the same pan.

To serve, fill the whole grain buns with the turkey burgers and grilled cherry tomatoes.

Benefits: The herb-infused turkey burgers provide lean proteins, while basil and mint have anti-inflammatory properties. Cherry tomatoes, rich in vitamin C and lycopene, have powerful antioxidant benefits.

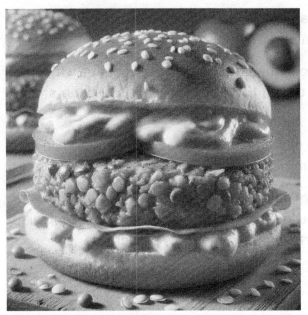

"Lentil and Vegetable Veggie Burgers with Avocado Sauce"

For 8 burgers:

400g of cooked lentils

2 large carrots, grated

1 small onion, chopped

2 garlic cloves, minced

1 red bell pepper, chopped

100g of gluten-free breadcrumbs

1 tablespoon of turmeric

Salt and pepper

8 gluten-free hamburger buns

For the avocado sauce:

2 ripe avocados

The juice of 1 lemon

1 tablespoon of extra virgin olive oil

Salt

Procedure: For the burgers, in a food processor, combine the lentils, carrots, onion, garlic, bell pepper, breadcrumbs, turmeric, salt, and pepper. Pulse until you get a homogeneous mixture.

Form 8 burgers and place them on a baking tray lined with parchment paper. Bake in a preheated oven at 200°C for 15-20 minutes or until golden.

Meanwhile, prepare the avocado sauce. In a bowl, mash the avocados with a fork until creamy. Add lemon juice, olive oil, and salt and stir until you get a smooth sauce.

To serve, split the hamburger buns in half and spread the avocado sauce on each half. Add the veggie burger and serve immediately.

Benefits: These lentil veggie burgers offer a wide range of anti-inflammatory nutrients, including fiber, plant-based proteins, and vitamins. Avocado provides healthy fats, while turmeric has powerful anti-inflammatory properties.

"Chickpea and Eggplant Veggie Burgers with Yogurt Sauce"

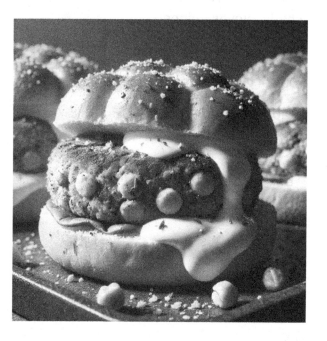

For 8 burgers:

400g of cooked chickpeas

1 large eggplant, grilled and chopped

1 small onion, chopped

2 garlic cloves, minced

100g of gluten-free breadcrumbs

1 tablespoon of cumin

Salt and pepper

8 gluten-free hamburger buns

For the yogurt sauce:

200g of Greek yogurt

1 garlic clove, minced

1 teaspoon of apple cider vinegar

Salt

Procedure: For the burgers, in a food processor, combine the chickpeas, grilled eggplant, onion, garlic, breadcrumbs, cumin, salt, and pepper. Pulse until you get a homogeneous mixture.

Form 8 burgers and place them on a baking tray lined with parchment paper. Bake in a preheated oven at 200°C for 15-20 minutes or until golden.

Meanwhile, prepare the yogurt sauce. In a bowl, combine the Greek yogurt, garlic, apple cider vinegar, and salt and stir until you get a smooth sauce.

To serve, split the hamburger buns in half and spread the yogurt sauce on each half. Add the veggie burger and serve immediately.

Benefits: The chickpea and eggplant veggie burgers are an excellent source of plant-based proteins and dietary fiber. The addition of cumin provides antioxidants and anti-inflammatory properties, while the Greek yogurt offers probiotics for gut health.

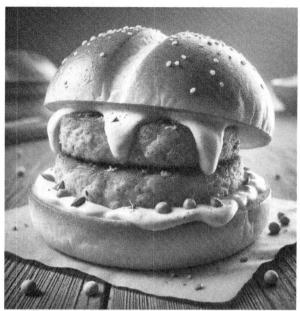

"Seitan Burgers Flavored with Tahini Sauce"

For 8 burgers:

500g of chopped seitan

2 tablespoons of soy sauce

1 teaspoon of turmeric

1 teaspoon of cumin

1 tablespoon of olive oil

Salt and pepper

8 hamburger buns

For the tahini sauce:

100g of tahini

Juice of 1 lemon

2 tablespoons of water

Salt

Procedure: Start by mixing the chopped seitan, soy sauce, turmeric, cumin, olive oil, salt, and pepper in a bowl. Stir well until you have a homogeneous mixture. Form 8 burgers.

Cook the burgers in a non-stick pan with a little oil for 3-4 minutes per side or until they are golden brown.

Meanwhile, prepare the tahini sauce. In a bowl, combine the tahini, lemon juice, water, and salt. Stir until you get a creamy sauce.

To serve, open the hamburger buns and spread the tahini sauce on each half. Add the seitan burger and serve immediately.

Benefits: The seitan burgers are a great source of plant proteins. The added turmeric and cumin are known for their anti-inflammatory properties. The tahini sauce provides a dose of healthy fats and calcium.

"Revolutionary Sandwiches"

"Sea Sandwich: The Embrace of the Ocean in a Bite"

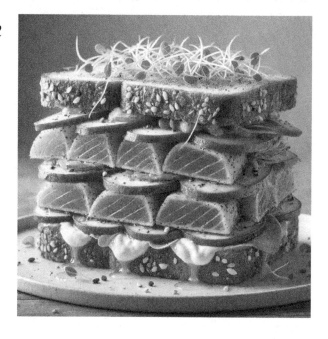

Ingredients for 4 people:

8 slices of whole wheat bread

300g of fresh tuna

2 ripe avocados

1 cucumber

200g of soy sprouts

4 tablespoons of Greek yogurt

Juice of one lemon

Extra virgin olive oil, salt, and pepper to taste

Procedure: Start by slicing the tuna thinly and quickly searing it in a pan with a drizzle of oil. Meanwhile, slice the avocado and cucumber thinly.

Once the tuna is ready, lightly toast the bread slices. In a bowl, mix the Greek yogurt with lemon juice, a pinch of salt, and pepper to obtain a fresh and light cream.

Now, assemble your sandwich: spread the yogurt cream on the bread, add slices of avocado, cucumber, soy sprouts, and finally the tuna. Top with another slice of bread and repeat the process for the remaining sandwiches.

Benefits: This "Sea Sandwich" is a true explosion of flavors and is rich in anti-inflammatory elements such as avocado, which is high in monounsaturated fatty acids, and tuna, a valuable source of Omega-3. Furthermore, with the contribution of vitamins and minerals from the cucumber and soy sprouts, this sandwich is a complete and balanced meal, perfect for a quick but healthy lunch.

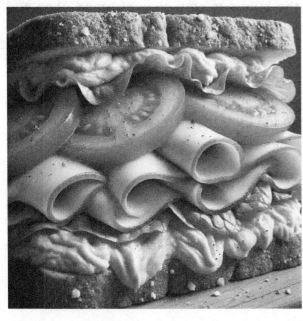

"Turquoise Sandwich: A Dive into Flavor with Turkey and Homemade Hummus"

Ingredients for 4 people:

For the hummus:

200g canned chickpeas

2 tablespoons of lemon juice

2 tablespoons of tahini

2 cloves of garlic

Extra virgin olive oil, salt, and pepper to taste

For the sandwich:

8 slices of whole wheat bread

400g of sliced turkey

2 ripe tomatoes

4 leaves of Romaine lettuce

Procedure: Start by preparing the hummus. Blend the chickpeas with lemon juice, tahini, garlic, salt, pepper, and a generous drizzle of olive oil until smooth. Season with salt and pepper to taste.

Meanwhile, slice the tomatoes and wash the lettuce leaves.

Lightly toast the bread slices. Spread the hummus on a slice of bread, then add lettuce, tomato slices, and finally the turkey slices. Top with another slice of bread and repeat for the other sandwiches.

Benefits: The "Turquoise Sandwich" is a true delight. Rich in protein from the turkey and with a homemade hummus cream that adds a unique taste note, it is also a valuable source of antioxidants thanks to the tomatoes. The lettuce provides fiber, contributing to a balanced and healthy meal. A sandwich that is a real treasure of well-being.

"Vegan Sphere Sandwich: An Explosion of Flavor with Seitan and Crunchy Vegetables"

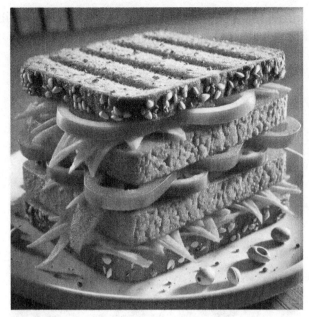

Ingredients for 4 people:

8 slices of multigrain bread

400g of seitan

1 red bell pepper

2 carrots

1 red onion

Extra virgin olive oil, salt, and pepper to taste

Sweet paprika to taste

Procedure: Start by slicing the seitan and cooking it in a pan with a drizzle of olive oil, a pinch of salt, pepper, and a sprinkle of paprika. Meanwhile, cut the bell pepper into strips, grate the carrots, and thinly slice the onion.

Toast the slices of multigrain bread. Then, on a slice of bread, place a portion of seitan, add the grated carrots, bell pepper strips, and onion slices. Top with another slice of bread and repeat for the other sandwiches.

Benefits: The "Vegan Sphere Sandwich" is a true delight for the palate. Its strength lies in the combination of protein-rich seitan and crunchy vegetables. This sandwich not only pleases with its unique flavor but also offers a wide range of health-beneficial nutrients. Rich in antioxidants from the carrots and bell peppers, it provides a significant dose of vitamins and fiber. A bite that combines the pleasure of taste with bodily well-being.

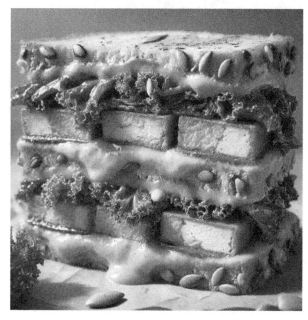

"Green Wizard Sandwich: The Charm of Tofu and Kale in a Pumpkin Sauce Embrace"

Ingredients for 4 people:

8 slices of seed bread

400g of tofu

200g of curly kale

1 small pumpkin

Fresh aromatic herbs (sage, thyme, rosemary)

Extra virgin olive oil, salt, and pepper to taste

Procedure: Start by slicing the tofu and cooking it in a pan with a drizzle of olive oil, a pinch of salt, and pepper. Meanwhile, clean and cube the pumpkin and steam it until soft. Blend the pumpkin with a drizzle of olive oil, salt, pepper, and the aromatic herbs until smooth.

In a pan, sauté the curly kale with a bit of oil and a pinch of salt until crispy.

Toast the slices of seed bread. Spread the pumpkin cream on a slice of bread, add the crispy kale, the slices of tofu, and top with another slice of bread. Repeat for the other sandwiches.

Benefits: The "Green Wizard Sandwich" is a journey of taste into the vegetarian world. Tofu provides a significant amount of protein, curly kale offers fiber and antioxidants, while the pumpkin cream enriches the sandwich with its sweet flavor and softness, bringing essential vitamins and minerals. A tasty and nutritious proposal, full of color and vitality.

"Wrap Wellness in a Bite"

"Eastern Embrace Wrap: Salmon Hug with Mango Sauce"

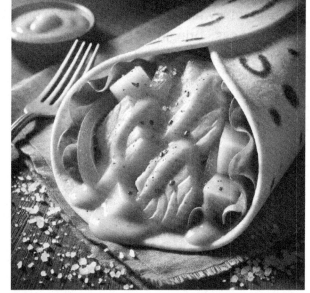

Ingredients for 4 people:

4 whole wheat tortillas

400g of fresh salmon

2 ripe mangoes

1 red bell pepper

Extra virgin olive oil, salt, and pepper to taste

Procedure: Begin by cutting the salmon into strips and cooking it in a pan with a drizzle of olive oil, a pinch of salt, and pepper. Meanwhile, clean and dice the mango and bell pepper. Blend the mango with a drizzle of olive oil, salt, and pepper until smooth to make a creamy sauce.

Briefly heat the tortillas in a non-stick pan, then spread them with the mango sauce. Add the salmon strips and diced bell pepper, then wrap the tortillas to form the wraps.

Benefits: The "Eastern Embrace Wrap" is a journey of taste into exotic flavors. Salmon provides a significant amount of protein and Omega-3, while the mango sauce enriches the wrap with its sweet and tropical flavor, contributing vitamin C and antioxidants. The red bell pepper adds crunchiness and an additional dose of vitamins. A tasty, nutritious, and colorful dish!

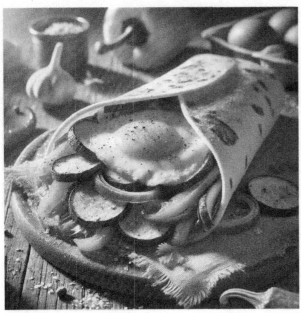

"Spring Wrap: A Meeting of Eggs and Crispy Vegetables"

Ingredients for 4 people:

4 corn of tortillas

4 large eggs

2 yellow bell peppers

2 small zucchinis

1 red onion

Extra virgin olive oil, salt, and pepper to taste

Procedure: Start by slicing the bell peppers, zucchinis, and red onion into thin strips. Sauté them in a pan with a drizzle of olive oil, salt, and pepper. Meanwhile, fry the eggs in a non-stick pan with a bit of oil.

Warm the tortillas in a non-stick pan, then spread them with the sautéed vegetables. Place a fried egg on top, then wrap the tortilla to form the wraps.

Benefits: The "Spring Wrap" is a symphony of fresh flavors and nutrients. Eggs provide high-quality protein, while the bell peppers, zucchinis, and onion supply fiber and vitamins. A mix that celebrates spring with its explosion of colors and flavors, packaged in a quick and healthy lunch. This wrap offers the perfect balance between nutrition and taste, making it an excellent option for an energizing meal at any time of the day.

"Forest Wraps: A Ballet of Porcini Mushrooms and Ricotta"

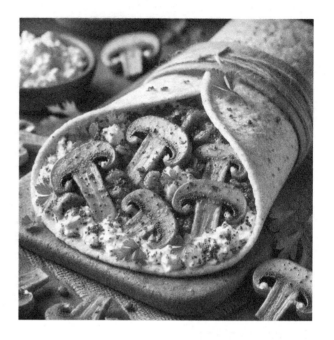

Ingredients for 4 people:

4 spelt tortillas

300g of fresh porcini mushrooms

2 cloves of garlic

Fresh parsley to taste

Extra virgin olive oil, salt, and pepper to taste

For the sauce:

200g of ricotta cheese

2 tablespoons of chopped parsley

Salt and pepper to taste

Procedure: Start by cleaning the porcini mushrooms and slicing them. In a pan, sauté the garlic in a drizzle of olive oil, then add the mushrooms. Sauté until they are golden and tender, then season with salt and pepper. Warm the tortillas in a non-stick pan.

For the sauce, blend the ricotta with parsley, adding a pinch of salt and pepper. The consistency should be creamy yet spreadable.

To assemble the wraps, lay out a tortilla and spread a quarter of the ricotta sauce in the center. Add a quarter of the sautéed porcini mushrooms and roll up the wrap. Repeat for the others.

Benefits: Tasting these "Forest Wraps" is like diving into an autumnal forest, where porcini mushrooms are the undisputed protagonists. The ricotta provides a touch of sweetness and creaminess, while the parsley adds a fresh note. This dish is a treasure trove of fiber and B vitamins, beneficial for the nervous and immune systems. A culinary experience that nourishes body and soul.

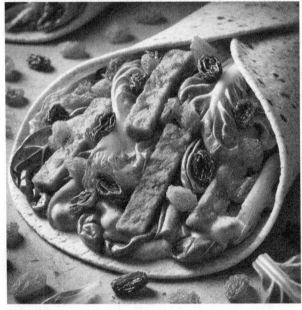

"Sunshine Wraps: Vegan Shades of Seitan and Escarole"

Ingredients for 4 people:

4 whole wheat tortillas

400g of seitan

1 head of escarole

2 tablespoons of raisins

Extra virgin olive oil, salt, and pepper to taste

For the sauce:

2 tablespoons of tahini

Juice of 1 lemon

2 tablespoons of water

Salt and pepper to taste

Procedure: Cut the seitan into strips and sauté in a pan with a drizzle of olive oil, salt, and pepper. Meanwhile, clean and chop the escarole, then add it to the seitan, cooking until wilted.

For the sauce, in a bowl, mix tahini, lemon juice, and water. Add salt and pepper to taste. The sauce should have a smooth and creamy consistency. Warm the tortillas in a non-stick pan.

To prepare the wraps, spread a quarter of the tahini sauce on a tortilla. Add a quarter of the seitan and escarole mix, then sprinkle with the raisins. Roll up the wrap and repeat for the others.

Benefits: With their nutritious and healthy ingredients, these "Sunshine Wraps" are a tasty and complete vegan dish. The raisins add a sweet touch, contrasting with the slight bitterness of the escarole, while the seitan provides quality plant-based proteins. The tahini, finally, offers a good dose of calcium and B vitamins. A dish that is a hymn to the sun and vitality.

Quote: *"The meal is not complete unless it ends with a dessert." - Oscar Wilde.*

CHAPTER 13:

"Desserts and Snacks: Responsible Pleasure"

We've arrived in the magical realm of responsible desserts and snacks, a world where indulgence marries health and pleasure combines with responsibility. This is the land of healthy delights, a place where appetite meets attention to well-being.

Imagine cheesecakes, elegant dancers twirling on the stage of your table, delightfully light yet nutritionally rich, or energizing bars, brimming with vitality for a tasty boost! Envision tartlets, small gems of flavor, deliciously fancy without the guilt of gluttony. And what about mousse? Sweet clouds that envelop you in an embrace of pleasure, while puddings and cupcakes, little heroes of comfort food, celebrate every moment with their delicious presence.

Then there are cookies, small travel companions that add a touch of sweetness to every moment, without ever forgetting the importance of conscious eating. And for a splash of freshness, let yourself be surprised by vegan milkshakes, a whirlwind of sweetness and nutrition.

This is the land of healthy delights, a paradise where indulgence is never a sin, but a right to enjoy life without compromising well-being.

"Healthy and Delicious Desserts: The Cheesecakes"

"Zen Cheesecake: The Anti-Inflammatory Triumph"

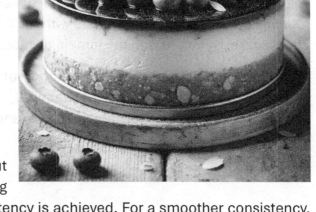

For the base:

200g of wholemeal biscuits

100g of almonds

80g of coconut butter (Coconut butter is easily made by blending coconut pulp until a creamy consistency is achieved. For a smoother consistency, strain the mixture. Store in the fridge. If coconut butter is not available, you can use coconut oil, which has a similar consistency when solid.)

For the cream:

500g of Greek yogurt

2 tablespoons of honey

The grated zest of 1 lemon

1 teaspoon of vanilla extract

3 sheets of gelatin

For the topping:

300g of blueberries (200g for preparation and 100 for garnish)

2 tablespoons of honey

Procedure: Begin by preparing the base. Blend the biscuits and almonds in a blender until they reach a breadcrumb-like consistency. Add the coconut butter and mix until smooth. Press the mixture into the bottom of a 24cm diameter cake tin and refrigerate for at least 30 minutes.

For the cream, whisk together the Greek yogurt, honey, lemon zest, and vanilla extract. Soak the gelatin in cold water for 10 minutes, squeeze out any excess water, and melt it in a saucepan with a little water until dissolved. Mix the gelatin with the yogurt and pour the mixture over the base. Refrigerate for at least 4 hours. For the topping, blend the 200g blueberries with the honey and spread the mixture over the cheesecake. Decorate with the remaining blueberries.

Benefits: "Zen Cheesecake" is a journey of well-being: blueberries are rich in antioxidants, lemon is a source of vitamin C, and almonds provide a good dose of vitamin E. A dessert that delights the palate and nourishes the body.

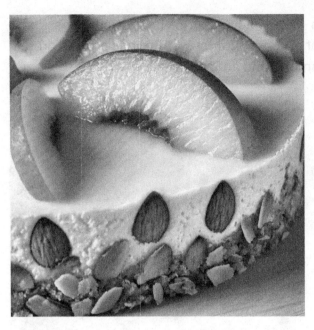

"Crunchy Delight: Almond and Peach Cheesecake"

For the base:

200g of almonds

100g of almond butter or lactose free butter

50g of Manuka honey

For the filling:

500g of Greek yogurt

3 organic eggs

200g of Manuka honey

1 teaspoon of vanilla extract

3 fresh peaches

Procedure: Begin by finely chopping the almonds and then mixing with the almond butter and honey. Spread this mixture into a 22 cm diameter baking tin to create the cheesecake base.

For the filling, beat together the Greek yogurt, eggs, honey, and vanilla extract until smooth. Slice the peaches thinly and gently fold them into the cream. Pour the mixture over the almond base.

Bake in a preheated oven at 180°C for about 1 hour or until the cheesecake is golden and cooked through. Allow to cool completely before serving.

Benefits: This cheesecake offers an incredible fusion of natural sweetness and crunchiness, with the added benefit of essential nutrients. Almonds provide protein and vitamin E, while peaches add vitamin C and antioxidants.

"Summer Dream: Cold Strawberry Cheesecake"

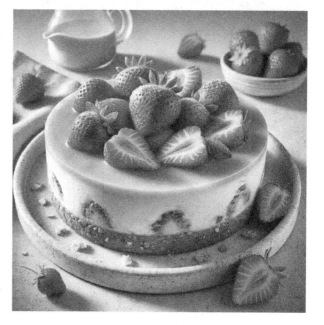

For the base:

200g of oat biscuits

100g of lactose-free butter

For the filling:

300g of fresh strawberries (200g for preparation and 100 for garnish)

200g of plant-based cream

100g of honey

2 tablespoons of powdered gelatin

Procedure: Begin by crushing the oat biscuits until they resemble breadcrumbs. Melt the butter and mix it with the crushed biscuits. Press the mixture into a 22 cm diameter cake tin to form the cheesecake base and refrigerate to set.

For the filling, place the 200g of strawberries, plant-based cream, and honey in a blender and blend until smooth. Dissolve the gelatin in a little hot water and then incorporate it into the strawberry mixture. Pour the filling over the biscuit base and refrigerate for at least 4 hours or until it has completely set. Decorate with the remaining strawberries.

Benefits: This cold cheesecake is a triumph of flavor and nutrition. Strawberries provide vitamin C, the plant-based cream offers a velvety consistency, and the oat biscuits add beneficial fiber.

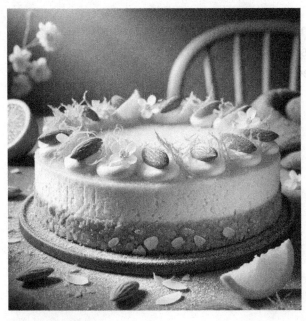

"Bittersweet Cheesecake: The Embrace of Citrus and Orange Blossoms"

For the base:

200g of oat biscuits

100g of lactose-free butter

For the filling:

500g of ricotta

200g of honey

4 eggs

Grated zest of 1 lemon and 1 orange

1 teaspoon of orange blossom essence

30g of toasted almonds

Procedure: For the base, grind the biscuits until they resemble breadcrumbs. Melt the butter and mix it with the ground biscuits. Press the mixture into a 22 cm diameter cake tin to form the cheesecake base and refrigerate to set.

For the filling, in a bowl combine the ricotta, honey, eggs, grated citrus zests, and orange blossom essence. Mix until smooth and homogeneous. Pour the filling over the base and level with a spatula.

Sprinkle the toasted almonds on top and bake in a preheated oven at 180°C for about 60 minutes or until the cheesecake is golden and firm to the touch. Allow to cool completely before unmolding.

Benefits: This cheesecake offers a symphony of flavors: the ricotta provides protein, the citrus vitamin C, and the almonds healthy fats and fiber. The orange blossom essence adds a refined and unexpected note.

"Velvety Desserts with Intense Flavors: Mousse and Puddings"

"Avocado Cocoa Mousse: A Flavorful Anti-inflammatory Dessert"

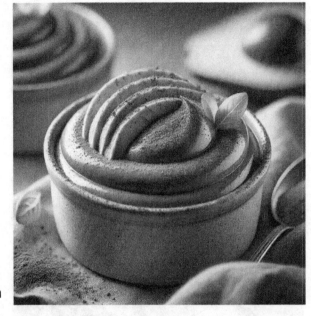

Ingredients for 4 servings:

2 ripe avocados

4 tablespoons of unsweetened cocoa powder

3 tablespoons of raw honey

2 tablespoons of coconut oil

1 teaspoon of vanilla extract

A pinch of salt

100 ml of almond milk

Procedure: Start by peeling the avocados and removing the pits. Place the avocado flesh in a blender along with the cocoa powder, honey, coconut oil, vanilla extract, salt, and almond milk. Blend everything until you achieve a smooth and homogeneous cream. Distribute the mousse into four small cups and refrigerate for at least two hours before serving.

Benefits: The "Avocado Cocoa Mousse" is more than just a dessert; it's a unique taste experience that takes care of your health. Rich in antioxidants from the cocoa, it provides healthy fats from the avocado and coconut oil, while the honey contributes its antibacterial and digestive properties. Finally, the almond milk adds a touch of sweetness and creaminess without weighing down the dessert.

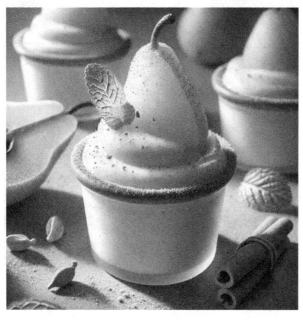

"Surprising Pear and Cardamom Mousse: An Elegant and Nutritious Dessert"

Ingredients for 4 servings:

3 ripe pears

200ml of plant-based cream

2 tablespoons of honey

1 teaspoon of ground cardamom

1 tablespoon of lemon juice

Mint leaves for garnishing

Procedure: Start by peeling the pears, removing the seeds, and cutting them into cubes. In a pot, combine the pears, honey, and cardamom. Cook over medium heat until the pears are soft, about 15-20 minutes. Cool the pear mixture slightly, then add the lemon juice and blend everything together. Whip the plant-based cream and fold it into the blended pears, mixing from the bottom up until smooth. Distribute the mousse into 4 cups and refrigerate for at least 2 hours before serving. Garnish with fresh mint leaves for a touch of color.

Benefits: This mousse offers a surprising union of fruity sweetness and spicy aroma. Pears are rich in vitamins, fiber, and antioxidants, while cardamom is known for its anti-inflammatory and digestive properties.

"Rice and Mango Pudding: A Sweet and Nutritious Dessert"

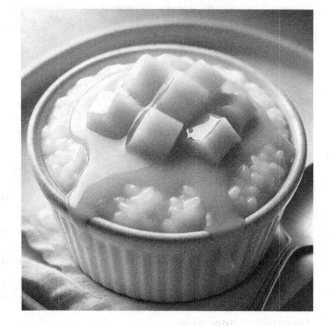

Ingredients for 4 servings:

1 liter of rice milk

100g of pudding rice

3 tablespoons of raw honey

1 ripe mango

Fresh mint leaves for garnish

Procedure: Begin by rinsing the rice under cold water, then place it in a pot with the rice milk. Bring to a boil, then reduce the heat and let it simmer slowly for 40-45 minutes, stirring often. Once the rice is cooked and the liquid has been absorbed, add the honey and mix well.

In the meantime, peel and dice the mango. Blend half of the mango until smooth to create a puree. Dice the other half for garnish.

Once the rice pudding has cooled slightly, distribute it into 4 bowls. Top with the mango puree and fresh mango cubes. Garnish with fresh mint leaves and serve.

Benefits: This pudding is a triumph of flavor and nutrition. The mango provides vitamins and antioxidants, the rice delivers slow-releasing carbohydrates, and the honey adds a touch of natural sweetness.

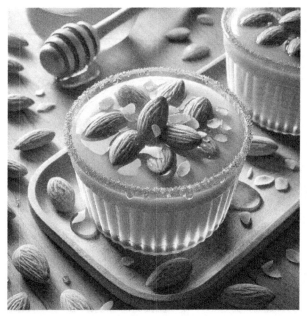

"Almond and Honey Pudding: A Healthy and Delicious Dessert"

Ingredients for 4 servings:

800ml of almond milk

4 tablespoons of honey

100g of almond flour

1 packet of agar agar

Toasted almond flakes for garnish

Procedure: Start by mixing the almond flour with a bit of almond milk until smooth. In a pot, bring the rest of the almond milk to a boil with the honey. Once boiling, reduce the heat and add the agar agar. Mix well to completely dissolve the agar agar.

Slowly add the almond paste to the boiling milk, continuing to stir to avoid lumps. Continue to simmer for 5-10 minutes, until the mixture has thickened.

Pour the pudding into bowls and let cool to room temperature. Once cooled, refrigerate for at least 2 hours. Before serving, garnish with toasted almond flakes.

Benefits: This almond pudding is a true jewel of nutrition. Almonds provide vitamin E and magnesium, while honey offers natural sweetness and antioxidants.

"Fragrant Soft-Hearted Treats: Tartlets"

"Summer Whole Wheat Tartlets with Yogurt Cream and Berries"

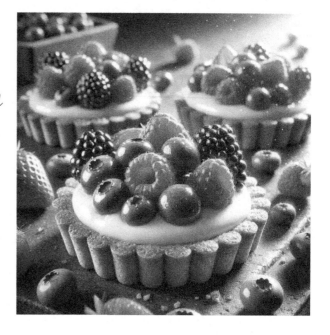

For 10 tartlets:

200g whole wheat flour

100g coconut butter

50g manuka honey

1 egg

A pinch of salt

For the yogurt cream:

500g Greek yogurt

2 tablespoons of honey

1 tablespoon of vanilla extract

Mixed berries (blueberries, blackberries, raspberries) for decoration

Procedure: Begin by mixing the whole wheat flour, coconut butter, honey, egg, and salt in a bowl. Work the ingredients until you have a homogeneous dough. Form a ball, wrap it in cling film, and let it rest in the refrigerator for 30 minutes.

Meanwhile, prepare the yogurt cream by mixing the Greek yogurt, honey, and vanilla extract in a bowl. Place it in the refrigerator until use.

Preheat the oven to 180°C. Roll out the dough and line 10 tartlet molds. Prick the bottom with a fork and bake in the oven for 15-20 minutes or until golden.

Once cooled, fill the tartlets with the yogurt cream and decorate with the berries. Serve immediately or store in the refrigerator until serving.

Benefits: These whole wheat tartlets with yogurt cream and berries are ideal for an afternoon break or as a dessert. Rich in fiber thanks to the whole wheat flour and antioxidants from the berries, they also provide a good source of protein from the yogurt.

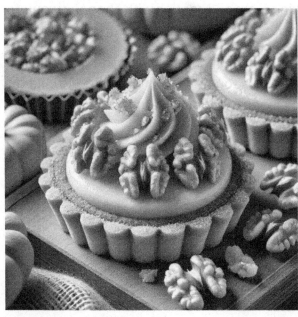

"Autumn Tartlets with Pumpkin Cream and Walnuts"

For 10 tartlets:

200g chestnut flour

100g lactose-free butter

50g maple syrup

1 egg

A pinch of salt

For the pumpkin cream:

500g pumpkin

50g coconut sugar

1 teaspoon cinnamon

Chopped walnuts for garnish

Procedure: Begin by mixing the chestnut flour, lactose-free butter, maple syrup, egg, and salt in a bowl. Work the ingredients until a uniform dough forms. Shape it into a ball, wrap in plastic, and refrigerate for 30 minutes.

Meanwhile, prepare the pumpkin cream. Steam the pumpkin until soft, then blend with coconut sugar and cinnamon until smooth.

Preheat the oven to 180°C (356°F). Roll out the dough and line 10 tartlet tins. Prick the bottom with a fork and bake for 15-20 minutes or until golden.

Once cooled, fill the tartlets with pumpkin cream and garnish with chopped walnuts. Serve immediately or store in the refrigerator until ready to serve.

Benefits: These autumn tartlets with pumpkin cream and walnuts are a true delight for the palate. The chestnut flour adds a rustic touch and is rich in fiber, while the pumpkin cream provides vitamin A, and cinnamon adds a warm autumnal aroma.

"Exquisite Tartlets with Chocolate Cream and Hazelnut Flour"

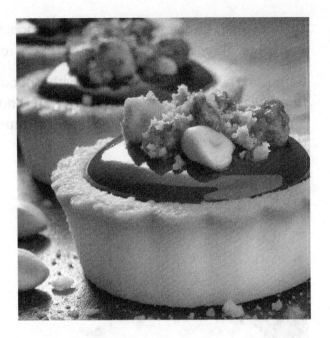

For 10 tartlets:

200g hazelnut flour

100g lactose-free butter

50g maple syrup

1 egg

A pinch of salt

For the chocolate cream:

200g 70% dark chocolate

200ml almond milk

2 tablespoons honey

Chopped hazelnuts for garnish

Procedure: Mix the hazelnut flour, lactose-free butter, maple syrup, egg, and salt in a bowl until a uniform dough forms. Shape into a ball, wrap in plastic, and refrigerate for 30 minutes.

Meanwhile, prepare the chocolate cream. Melt the chocolate in a double boiler, add almond milk and honey, and stir until smooth.

Preheat the oven to 180°C (356°F). Roll out the dough and line 10 tartlet tins. Prick the bottom with a fork and bake for 15-20 minutes or until golden.

Once cooled, fill the tartlets with the chocolate cream and garnish with chopped hazelnuts. Serve immediately or store in the refrigerator until ready to serve.

Benefits: These "Exquisite Tartlets with Chocolate Cream and Hazelnut Flour" are a true delight for the palate. Hazelnut flour and dark chocolate provide a generous dose of antioxidants, while honey adds a natural sweet aroma.

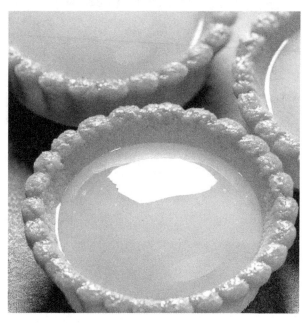

"Shining Lemon-Scented Tartlets"

For 10 tartlets:

200g almond flour

100g lactose-free butter

50g agave syrup

1 egg

A pinch of salt

For the lemon cream:

2 organic lemons

150g brown sugar

3 eggs

100g lactose-free butter

Procedure: Mix the almond flour, lactose-free butter, agave syrup, egg, and salt in a bowl until a uniform dough forms. Shape into a ball, wrap in plastic, and refrigerate for 30 minutes.

For the lemon cream, grate the zest of the lemons and squeeze the juice. Mix the juice and zest with brown sugar in a saucepan. Add eggs and butter and cook in a double boiler, stirring until it thickens.

Preheat the oven to 180°C (356°F). Roll out the dough and line 10 tartlet molds. Prick the bottom with a fork and bake for 15-20 minutes or until golden.

Once cooled, fill the tartlets with the lemon cream. Serve immediately or store in the refrigerator until ready to serve.

Benefits: These "Shining Lemon-Scented Tartlets" blend the sweetness of almond flour with the tanginess of lemons. Lemon, rich in vitamin C and antioxidants, is a perfect ingredient for a healthy sweet break.

"Delicious Treats: The Cupcakes"

"Soft Dream Cupcakes: Lemon & Poppy Seed Delights"

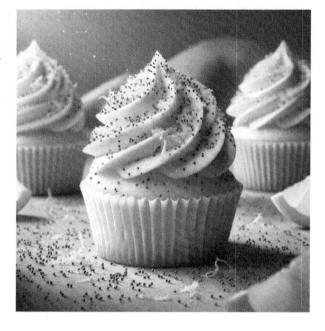

For 10 cupcakes:

200g whole wheat flour

2 teaspoons of baking powder

150g honey

100g melted coconut butter

3 eggs

Zest and juice of 2 lemons

2 tablespoons of poppy seeds

For the frosting:

200g light cream cheese

50g honey

Zest and juice of 1 lemon

Procedure: Start by preheating the oven to 180°C (356°F) and preparing a cupcake pan with 10 paper liners.

In a bowl, combine the flour, baking powder, lemon zest, and poppy seeds. In another bowl, whisk together the honey, melted coconut butter, eggs, and lemon juice. Combine the two mixtures and stir until you have a uniform batter.

Distribute the batter among the liners and bake for 20-25 minutes, or until the cupcakes are golden and a toothpick inserted into the center comes out clean. Allow to cool completely.

For the frosting, whisk together the cream cheese, honey, lemon juice, and zest. Spread the frosting over the cooled cupcakes.

Benefits: The "Soft Dream Cupcakes" are a treasure trove of antioxidants, thanks to the lemon and poppy seeds, while the honey provides natural sweetness. This delight offers a tasty way to enjoy a sweet yet healthy recipe.

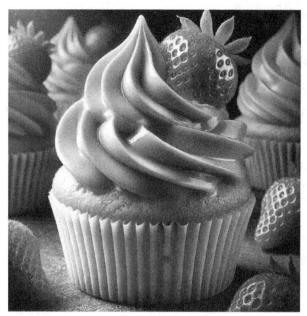

"Celestial Cupcakes: Strawberry & Luscious Cream"

For 10 cupcakes:

200g oat flour

1 teaspoon of baking powder

100g acacia honey

80g melted coconut oil

3 eggs

100g fresh strawberries, chopped

For the luscious cream:

200g light cream cheese

50g acacia honey

100g fresh strawberries, blended

Procedure: Preheat the oven to 180°C (356°F) and prepare a cupcake pan with 10 paper liners.

In a bowl, combine the oat flour, baking powder, and chopped strawberries. In another bowl, whisk together the honey, coconut oil, and eggs. Add the wet ingredients to the dry ingredients and stir until you have a uniform batter.

Distribute the batter among the liners and bake for 20-25 minutes, or until golden. Allow to cool completely.

For the cream, whip the cream cheese with the honey and blended strawberries. Once the cupcakes have cooled, spread the luscious cream on top.

Benefits: These cupcakes are a burst of antioxidants, thanks to the strawberries, while the oat flour and acacia honey contribute to providing natural sweetness. This recipe is for those who love sweets but aim to maintain a healthy diet.

"*Paradisiacal Cupcakes: Coconut & Exotic Fruit*"

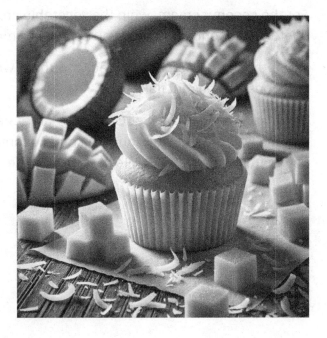

For 10 cupcakes:

200g coconut flour

1 teaspoon of baking soda

100g raw honey

80g melted coconut oil

3 eggs

100g exotic fruit (papaya, pineapple, mango), chopped

For the coconut cream:

50g coconut flour

200g vegetable cream

50g raw honey

Toasted coconut flakes for decoration

Procedure: Preheat the oven to 180°C (356°F) and prepare a cupcake pan with 10 paper liners.

In a bowl, combine the coconut flour, baking soda, and chopped exotic fruit. In another bowl, whisk together the honey, coconut oil, and eggs. Mix the wet ingredients into the dry ingredients until you have a uniform batter.

Distribute the batter among the liners and bake for 20-25 minutes, or until golden. Allow to cool completely.

For the coconut cream, whip the vegetable cream with the honey, then incorporate it into the coconut flour until you achieve a smooth cream.

Once the cupcakes have cooled, top them with the coconut cream and decorate with toasted coconut flakes.

Benefits: The Paradisiacal Cupcakes are a celebration of antioxidants, fiber, and vitamin C, thanks to the exotic fruit and coconut. A heavenly dessert that transports you to tropical beaches while keeping your health a priority.

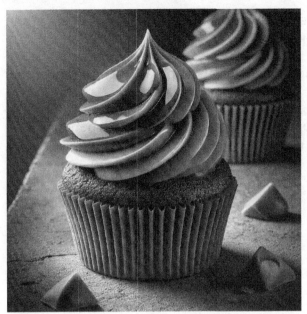

"Emotion Cupcake: Chocolate & Hazelnut Cream"

For 10 cupcakes:

100g whole wheat flour

25g unsweetened cocoa powder

1 teaspoon of baking soda

2 eggs

70g melted coconut oil

85g acacia honey

50g almond milk

For the hazelnut cream:

200g hazelnut flour

2 tablespoons acacia honey

1 tablespoon extra-virgin olive oil

A pinch of sea salt

Procedure: Preheat the oven to 180°C (356°F) and prepare a cupcake tray with 10 paper liners.

In a bowl, combine the whole wheat flour, cocoa, and baking soda. In another bowl, whisk together the eggs, coconut oil, honey, and almond milk. Mix the wet ingredients into the dry ingredients until you have a uniform batter.

Distribute the batter among the liners and bake for 20-25 minutes, or until a toothpick inserted comes out clean. Allow to cool completely.

For the hazelnut cream, blend the hazelnut flour, honey, olive oil, and a pinch of salt in a blender until you achieve a smooth and silky cream.

Once the cupcakes have completely cooled, generously spread the hazelnut cream on the surface.

Benefits: This recipe combines the pleasure of sweetness with health benefits. Rich in vitamin E, good fats, and fiber, these treats offer a delicious flavor while contributing to overall well-being.

"Snacks: Nutrition at the Right Time: The Cookies"

"Morning Friends Cookies: Soft Coconut & Lime"

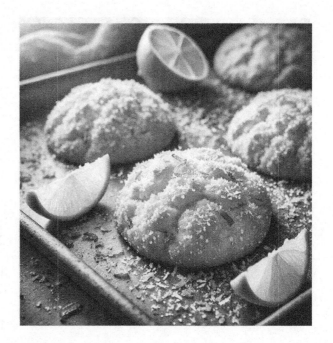

Recipe for about 15/20 cookies:

200g coconut flour

80g melted coconut oil

100g acacia honey

Grated zest and juice of 1 lime

1 teaspoon baking soda

2 eggs

Procedure: Preheat the oven to 180°C and line a baking sheet with parchment paper. In a bowl, mix the coconut flour, coconut oil, honey, lime zest, lime juice, and baking soda. In another bowl, beat the eggs, then add them to the coconut mixture and mix until a uniform dough is formed.

Take small portions of dough and, with your hands, shape them into discs about 4 cm in diameter. Place them on the prepared baking sheet, making sure to leave space between them.

Bake for 10-12 minutes, or until the cookies are slightly golden. Allow them to cool completely on the baking sheet before transferring to a wire rack to cool completely.

Benefits: The Morning Friends Cookies are an energetic and anti-inflammatory boost. Rich in fiber and beneficial fatty acids, they provide satiety and well-being. Lime, a source of vitamin C, refreshes the palate and enhances immune defenses.

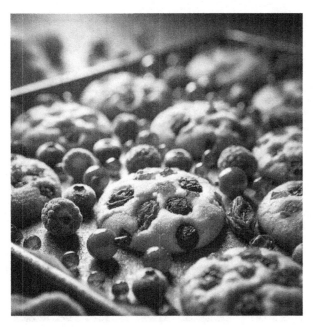

"Aurora Borealis Cookies: Hazelnut & Red Berry Cookies"

Recipe for about 15/20 cookies:

200g hazelnut flour

100g dried red berries (blueberries, raspberries, currants)

100g acacia honey

80g extra virgin olive oil

1 egg

1 teaspoon vanilla extract

1 teaspoon baking soda

A pinch of salt

Procedure: Preheat the oven to 180°C and line a baking sheet with parchment paper. In a large bowl, combine the hazelnut flour, red berries, baking soda, and salt. In another bowl, whisk together the olive oil, egg, honey, and vanilla extract until smooth.

Mix the wet ingredients into the dry ingredients until a cohesive dough forms. Using a spoon, scoop portions of the dough onto the baking sheet, spacing them apart.

Bake for 15-20 minutes, or until the cookies are golden. Allow them to cool completely on the baking sheet before transferring to a wire rack to cool completely.

Benefits: These cookies are an explosion of flavors and nutrients. Rich in fiber, vitamins, and antioxidants, they are the perfect choice for a sweet and nutritious break.

"Spiced Exotic Cookies: Almond & Spice Cookies"

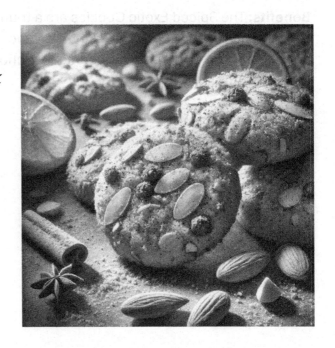

Recipe for about 15/20 cookies:

200g whole wheat flour

100g chopped almonds

1 teaspoon cinnamon

1/2 teaspoon nutmeg

1/4 teaspoon ground cloves

100g raw honey

1 egg

80g extra virgin olive oil

1 teaspoon baking soda

Grated zest of 1 organic orange

Procedure: Preheat the oven to 180°C and line a baking sheet with parchment paper. In a bowl, mix the whole wheat flour, chopped almonds, cinnamon, nutmeg, cloves, baking soda, and orange zest. In another bowl, whisk together the egg, honey, and olive oil.

Combine the wet ingredients with the dry ingredients and mix until a uniform dough forms. Shape the dough into discs about 3cm in diameter and place them on the baking sheet.

Bake the cookies for 15-20 minutes, until they are golden. Let them cool completely on the baking sheet before removing them.

Benefits: The Spiced Exotic Cookies are a triumph of flavors and aromas. Thanks to the presence of spices such as cinnamon and nutmeg, they offer anti-inflammatory and antioxidant benefits. The addition of chopped almonds provides a valuable source of protein and fiber.

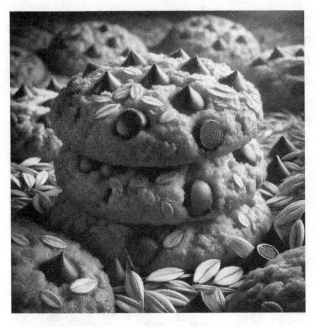

"Golden Sunset Cookies: Oat & Dark Chocolate Chips Cookies"

Recipe for about 15/20 cookies:

200g oat flour

100g dark chocolate chips

80g almond butter or lactose free butter

70g raw honey

1 egg

1 teaspoon baking soda

A pinch of sea salt

Procedure: Preheat the oven to 180°C and line a baking sheet with parchment paper. In a large bowl, combine the oat flour, dark chocolate chips, baking soda, and sea salt. In another bowl, whisk together the almond butter, egg, and honey until smooth.

Combine the wet ingredients with the dry ingredients and mix until a cohesive dough forms. Using a spoon, scoop portions of the dough and place them on the baking sheet in spaced-out mounds.

Bake for 12-15 minutes, or until the cookies are golden. Let them cool completely on the baking sheet before transferring them to a wire rack to cool down completely.

Benefits: The Golden Sunset Cookies blend the sweetness of chocolate with the rustic texture of oats, in a perfect mix of flavor and health. Rich in fiber and antioxidants, they provide energy and balance throughout the day.

"Autumn Whispers Cookies: Soft Apple & Cinnamon"

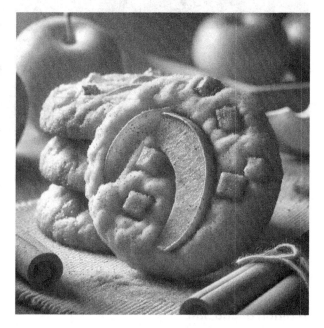

Recipe for about 15/20 cookies:

200g whole wheat flour

2 medium-sized apples

80g olive oil

100g brown sugar

2 teaspoons ground cinnamon

1 teaspoon baking powder

2 eggs

Procedure: Preheat the oven to 180°C and line a baking tray with parchment paper. Peel and grate the apples, then cut them into small cubes. In a bowl, combine the flour, brown sugar, cinnamon, and baking powder. In another bowl, whisk the eggs with the oil, then add this mixture to the dry ingredients. Also, add the diced apples and stir until you get a uniform dough.

Using a spoon, take some of the dough and form discs on the prepared tray, leaving space between them. Bake for 15-20 minutes, or until the cookies are golden. Let them cool completely on the tray before transferring them to a rack to cool down completely.

Benefits: These cookies are a delight that combines taste and health. Rich in fiber thanks to the whole wheat flour and apples, they contribute to a healthy sense of fullness. Olive oil provides healthy fats, while cinnamon offers antioxidant and anti-inflammatory properties. Lastly, brown sugar is a natural sweetener, a healthier alternative to refined sugar. These cookies are the perfect way to start the day or for an afternoon snack.

"Every Bite is a Surprise: Homemade Energy Bars"

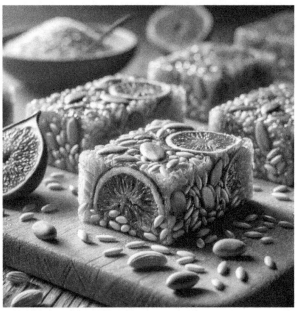

"Sunshine Bars: The Flavor Explosion of Wheat Sprouts"

Recipe for 15/20 bars:

200g of dried figs

150g of sunflower seeds

100g of wheat sprouts

50g of acacia honey

40g of sesame seeds

30g of extra virgin olive oil

1 tablespoon of fresh lemon juice

A pinch of sea salt

Procedure: Place the dried figs in a bowl and cover with hot water. Let them soak for 10 minutes, then drain and set aside.

In a blender, combine the sunflower seeds, wheat sprouts, honey, sesame seeds, olive oil, lemon juice, and sea salt. Add the soaked dried figs and blend until the mixture comes together.

Line a rectangular baking tray with parchment paper. Spread the mixture evenly, pressing down firmly to compact it. Refrigerate for at least 2 hours.

Once chilled, cut the mixture into 15/20 bars and store in an airtight container in the fridge.

Benefits: Sunshine Bars are a source of energy, protein, and fiber thanks to the sunflower seeds and wheat sprouts. The sweet and natural taste of figs perfectly complements the crunchiness of the seeds, making them an irresistible and healthy snack.

"Eastern Light Energy Bars: Almonds & Goji Berries"

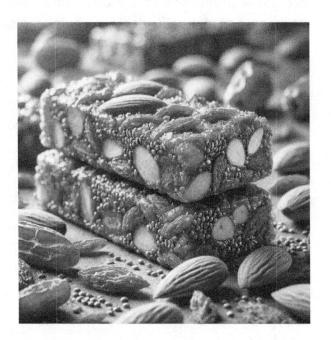

Recipe for 15/20 bars:

150g whole almonds

100g goji berries

100g Medjool dates, pitted

50g chia seeds

50g acacia honey

30g coconut oil, melted

Zest of 1 organic orange

1 teaspoon ground cinnamon

Procedure: Place the dates in a bowl and cover with hot water. Let them soak for 10 minutes, then drain and set aside.

In a blender, combine almonds, goji berries, chia seeds, honey, coconut oil, orange zest, and cinnamon. Add the soaked dates and blend until you get a uniform mixture.

Line a rectangular baking tray with parchment paper. Spread the mixture evenly, pressing down firmly to compact. Refrigerate for at least 2 hours.

Once chilled, cut the mixture into 15/ 20 bars and store in an airtight container in the fridge.

Benefits: These bars combine the antioxidant virtues of goji berries with the beneficial properties of almonds and chia seeds. A concentration of energy, vitamins, and minerals, ideal for a quick replenishment during the day.

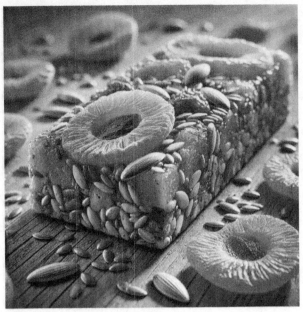

"Sunshine Energy Bars: Apricots & Sunflower Seeds"

Recipe for 15/20 bars:

200g dried apricots

100g sunflower seeds

50g flax seeds

50g acacia honey

40g extra virgin olive oil

Zest of 1 organic lemon

1 teaspoon ground vanilla

Procedure: Soak the dried apricots in warm water for 10 minutes. Drain them and set aside.

In a blender, combine the soaked apricots, sunflower seeds, flax seeds, honey, olive oil, lemon zest, and vanilla. Blend until you get a smooth paste.

Line a square baking tray with parchment paper. Spread the mixture evenly, pressing down carefully to compact it. Refrigerate for at least 2 hours.

After chilling, cut the mixture into 15/20 bars. Store in an airtight container in the fridge.

Benefits: Sunshine Energy Bars combine the sweet and refreshing taste of dried apricots with the crunch of sunflower and flax seeds for a burst of energy, fibers, and vitamins. A delicious snack that satisfies and benefits health.

"Hazelnut & Cocoa Energy Bars"

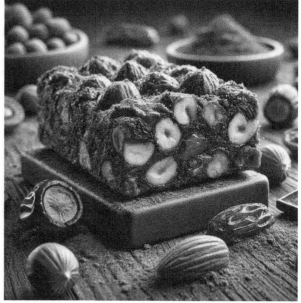

Recipe for 15/20 bars:

200g of dried dates

150g of hazelnut flour

50g of unsweetened cocoa powder

100g of acacia honey

50g of extra virgin olive oil

Procedure: Soak the dates in hot water for 10 minutes, then drain and dry them.

In a blender, combine the soaked dates, hazelnut flour, cocoa, honey, and oil. Blend until you get a uniform dough.

Line a rectangular pan with parchment paper and spread the mixture, pressing it down well with your hands or the back of a spoon.

Refrigerate for at least 2 hours. Once thoroughly chilled, cut the bars and store them in an airtight container in the refrigerator.

Benefits: These bars are a perfect blend of taste and health. Cocoa, rich in antioxidants, and hazelnuts, a source of good fats, create a delicious snack that provides energy and nourishes the body.

"Indulgent Snack: Vegan Milkshakes"

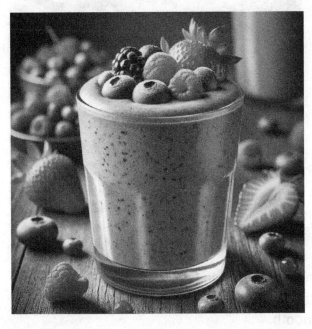

"Gourmet Vegan Milkshake: A Burst of Berry Freshness"

For 1 serving, you will need:

1 cup of mixed berries (strawberries, blueberries, raspberries)

1 ripe banana

1 cup of unsweetened oat milk

1 tablespoon of flaxseeds

4-5 ice cubes

Procedure: Gather your berries and banana in the blender, add the oat milk. Blend everything until smooth. Then, add the flaxseeds and ice cubes, and blend again until the milkshake reaches a delightfully creamy and refreshing consistency.

Here's your Gourmet Vegan Milkshake with Mixed Berries! A vitamin and antioxidant cocktail that will offer you a moment of delightful freshness.

Benefits: Berries are a true goldmine of antioxidants, perfect for fighting inflammation. Flaxseeds provide a dose of fibers and omega-3, while oat milk enriches it all with a delicate and nutritious flavor. This milkshake is a fresh and healthy embrace!

"Ray of Sunshine: Vegan Peach and Ginger Milkshake"

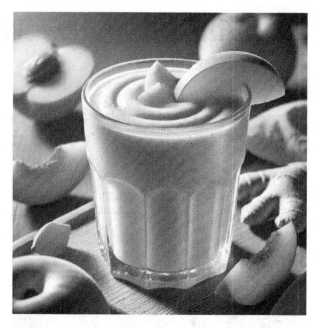

For 1 serving, you will need:

2 ripe peaches

1 cm of fresh ginger root

1 cup of unsweetened almond milk

1 teaspoon of acacia honey (or agave syrup for a completely vegan option)

4-5 ice cubes

Procedure: Start by peeling the peaches and removing the pits, then cut them into pieces and place them in the blender. Add the peeled piece of ginger root and the almond milk. Blend everything until smooth.

Then, add the honey or agave syrup and the ice cubes, and blend again until the milkshake reaches the desired consistency, creamy and refreshing.

Benefits: A true dive into summer freshness! Peaches, sweet and juicy, provide a rich dose of vitamins A and C, while ginger adds a spicy touch that stimulates digestion. Almond milk contributes with plant proteins and a touch of sweetness, making this milkshake an excellent choice for a refreshing and healthy snack.

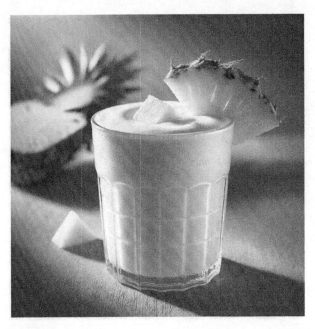

"Dreamy Tropical: Vegan Pineapple and Coconut Milk Milkshake"

For 1 serving, you will need:

1 cup of fresh pineapple cubes

1 cup of unsweetened coconut milk

1 tablespoon of agave syrup or honey (for a fully vegan option, use agave syrup)

4-5 ice cubes

Procedure: Begin by placing the fresh pineapple cubes in the blender. Add the coconut milk and blend until smooth. Then, add the agave syrup or honey and the ice cubes, and blend again until the milkshake becomes creamy and cold.

Benefits: The "Dreamy Tropical" is an exotic journey in a sip! Pineapple, rich in vitamin C and bromelain, an enzyme that aids digestion, wonderfully combines with the creaminess of coconut milk, which provides healthy fats and a touch of tropical flavor. This milkshake is an ideal choice for a summer refreshment or an afternoon snack, offering a balanced mix of natural sweetness, vital nutrients, and delightful freshness.

"Chocolate Paradise: Vegan Cocoa and Almond Milk Milkshake"

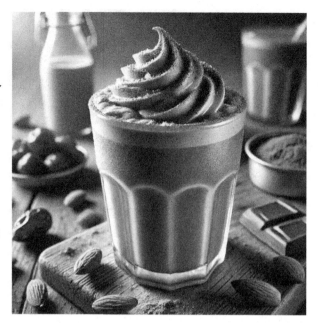

For 1 serving, you will need:

2 tablespoons of unsweetened cocoa powder

1 cup of unsweetened almond milk

2 Medjool dates, pitted

4-5 ice cubes

Procedure: Place the pitted dates in the blender and blend until they become a paste. Add the cocoa powder and almond milk. Blend until you achieve a smooth and creamy consistency. Finally, add the ice cubes and blend again until the milkshake becomes deliciously cold.

Benefits: The "Chocolate Paradise" is an indulgent yet healthy milkshake. The abundance of cocoa provides an antioxidant boost and a deep chocolate flavor, while the dates offer natural sweetness and a dose of fiber. The almond milk adds a creamy texture and a delicate flavor, perfectly complementing the intensity of the cocoa. It's a milkshake that not only satisfies the palate but also nourishes the body. A true guilty pleasure, without the guilt!

Quote: *"You cannot think well, love well, sleep well, if you have not eaten well." - Virginia Woolf.*

CHAPTER 14

"The Elegance of Gourmet Flavor"

Creating Anti-Inflammatory Gourmet Recipes is a fascinating culinary journey where gastronomic excellence meets bodily well-being. There's an undeniable refinement in balancing complex flavors, aesthetic presentation, and health benefits. This is the true heart of gourmet culinary art, and in this chapter, we take it a step further.

Preparing gourmet dishes that fight inflammation isn't just an exercise culinary skill but also an act of care towards ourselves and our loved ones. Each dish is an invitation to enjoy a complete sensory experience that not only satisfies the palate but also nourishes the body and promotes health. In this journey, we will discover how the elegance of flavor can truly embrace our aspiration for well-being.

Let's get ready to dive into a world where cooking becomes a perfect fusion of art and science. A world where food, far from being a mere necessity or pleasure, transforms into a powerful tool for health. We are ready to embrace this challenge with enthusiasm, to learn, experiment, and create. Let's prepare to unveil the elegance of flavor in all its forms, in this exciting gourmet journey into anti-inflammatory eating.

"A Triumph of Taste and Health: Gourmet Appetizers"

In this culinary world where elegance meets health, the art of cooking blends with nutritional experimentation, creating an enchanting crossroad that elevates both the table and the body's well-being. Each appetizer is a celebration of complex flavors and seductive nuances, crafted for the pleasure of the senses and to promote health.

In every appetizer, there's a dialogue between ingredients, a conversation of flavors that enhance each other in perfect balance. There's a deep respect for every single ingredient, valuing its role and its contribution to the final dish. It's an approach to eating that goes beyond mere nutrition, transforming it into an aesthetic and emotional experience. It's a hymn to the joy of eating healthily and the triumph of a cuisine that celebrates both taste and health.

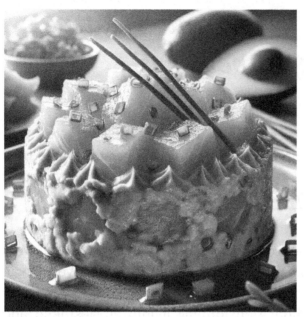

"Royal Appetizer: Salmon Tartare with Avocado and Ginger"

Ingredients for 4 people:

400g of fresh salmon

2 ripe avocados

1 teaspoon of grated fresh ginger

Juice of 1 lime

Sea salt and freshly ground black pepper to taste

1 tablespoon of extra virgin olive oil

Chives for garnish

Procedure: Start by dicing the salmon into small cubes and place it in a bowl. Add the grated fresh ginger, lime juice, extra virgin olive oil, salt, and pepper. Mix gently and let marinate in the refrigerator for 15 minutes.

Meanwhile, cut the avocados in half, remove the pit, and scoop out the flesh with a spoon. Mash them with a fork until creamy and season with salt and pepper.

Take four plates and place a pastry ring in the center. Fill it halfway with the avocado cream and then with the marinated salmon. Gently remove the ring and garnish with chopped chives. Repeat for all the plates.

Benefits: "The Royal Appetizer" offers a unique blend of flavors and health benefits. Salmon and avocado, rich in Omega 3, contribute to cardiovascular health, while ginger acts as a powerful anti-inflammatory. A gourmet and healthy start to the meal."

"Stellar Appetizer: Red Beet Carpaccio with Goat Cheese and Pumpkin Seeds"

Ingredients for 4 people:

4 medium red beets

200g goat cheese

2 tablespoons pumpkin seeds

1 tablespoon balsamic vinegar

2 tablespoons extra virgin olive oil

Salt and freshly ground black pepper to taste

Chives for garnishing

Procedure: Preheat the oven to 180°C (356°F). Wrap the beets in aluminum foil and bake for about an hour, or until tender. Allow to cool, then peel and slice thinly.

Toast the pumpkin seeds in a dry pan until they turn golden and start to pop.

Prepare a dressing with balsamic vinegar, extra virgin olive oil, salt, and pepper.

Arrange the beet slices on four plates, sprinkle with crumbled goat cheese and toasted pumpkin seeds. Drizzle with the prepared dressing and garnish with chopped chives.

Benefits: This appetizer combines the earthy flavor of red beets, the creaminess of goat cheese, and the crunch of pumpkin seeds, creating a unique gastronomic experience. Rich in antioxidants and fiber, this appetizer helps promote digestive health.

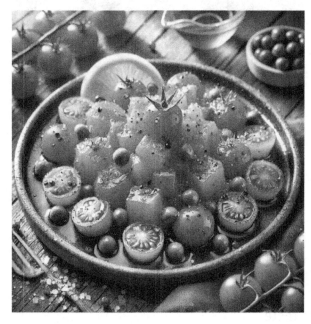

"Mediterranean Gourmet Appetizer: Tuna Tartare with Cherry Tomatoes and Capers"

Ingredients for 4 people:

400g fresh tuna

200g cherry tomatoes

2 tablespoons capers

2 tablespoons extra virgin olive oil

Juice of 1 lemon

Salt and freshly ground black pepper to taste

Fresh parsley for garnishing

Procedure: Cut the tuna into small cubes and place it in a bowl. Wash the cherry tomatoes, dry them, and cut them in half. Add the tomatoes and capers to the tuna.

In a small bowl, mix the olive oil, lemon juice, salt, and pepper. Pour this dressing over the tuna tartare, mixing well to blend all the ingredients.

Allow the mixture to rest in the refrigerator for at least 30 minutes before serving, so the flavors have time to meld perfectly. When serving, garnish with chopped fresh parsley.

Benefits: "The Mediterranean Tuna Tartare" is a dish rich in Omega-3, vitamin C, and lycopene. This refined combination, besides being extremely tasty, is a true concentration of health and well-being.

"Appetizer: Trout and Mango Rolls on a Bed of Arugula"

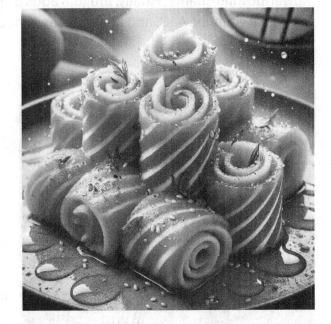

Ingredients for 4 people:

2 fresh trout fillets

1 ripe mango

100 grams of fresh arugula

Juice of 1 lemon

2 tablespoons extra virgin olive oil

Salt and pepper to taste

Sesame seeds for garnish

Procedure: Start with the trout. Remove the skin and cut the fillets into thin strips. Season with lemon juice, a pinch of salt, and pepper, and leave to marinate in the refrigerator for 15-20 minutes.

In the meantime, peel the mango and cut it into thin strips. Once the trout is ready, wrap each trout strip around a strip of mango, creating rolls.

To serve, arrange a bed of fresh arugula on the plates, place the trout and mango rolls on top, season with a drizzle of extra virgin olive oil, and garnish with sesame seeds.

Benefits: This appetizer is an explosion of flavors and nutrients. Trout is rich in omega-3, proteins, and B vitamins, important for heart and brain health. The mango adds a sweet and tropical touch to the dish and is rich in vitamins A and C, both powerful antioxidants. Finally, arugula adds a spicy and crunchy touch and is a good source of vitamins A, C, and K, as well as various minerals.

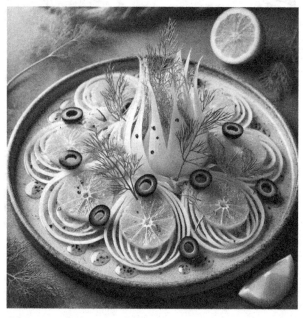

"Appetizer Elegance: Fennel and Orange Carpaccio"

Ingredients for 4 people:

2 large fennel bulbs

2 oranges

60g pitted black olives

1 lemon (juice and zest)

2 tablespoons extra virgin olive oil

Salt and fresh ground black pepper to taste

Fresh dill for garnish

Procedure: Wash and clean the fennels, then slice them very thinly using a mandoline or a sharp knife. Peel the oranges with a sharp knife, removing all the white part as well. Slice the oranges into thin slices. In a large bowl, mix the lemon juice and zest, extra virgin olive oil, salt, and pepper to create a dressing.

Add the fennel and orange slices to the dressing, gently mixing to ensure all the ingredients are well coated. Arrange the fennel and orange salad on four plates, sprinkle with the black olives, and garnish with fresh dill.

Benefits: "The Appetizer Elegance" is a symphony of fresh and vibrant flavors that come together in a mix of crunchiness and sweetness. Fennel and orange are rich in vitamin C and fiber, contributing to support the immune system and digestive health.

"A Symphony of Culinary Elegance: Gourmet First Courses"

Picture a garden blooming with splendid roses, an ensemble of colors, aromas, and shapes that blend into a harmonious and captivating painting. Just as a gardener nurtures each rose, so is every recipe cultivated with care, patience, and dedication.

Here, each dish is like a rare and precious rose, the result of careful selection and constant care. It's not just about growing ingredients, but about making them blossom into unique combinations, creating bouquets of flavors that delight the palate.

The kitchen here transforms into a lush garden, where every recipe is a flower blooming, revealing its colors, its fragrance, its unique flavor. It's a place where love for food, passion for health, and respect for nature are cultivated. In this culinary garden, the beauty of life is celebrated in every nuance.

"First Course: Gourmet Fettuccine with Truffle and Cranberries"

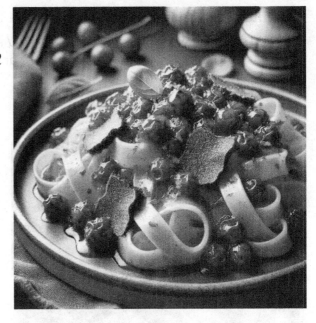

Ingredients for 4 people:

400g whole wheat fettuccine

30g black truffle

150g fresh cranberries

2 cloves of garlic

Extra virgin olive oil

Salt and pepper to taste

A pinch of nutmeg

Fresh basil leaves for garnish

Procedure: Boil a pot of salted water for the pasta. Meanwhile, in a non-stick pan, sauté the garlic cloves in extra virgin olive oil until golden, then remove them.

Add the cranberries to the pan and cook over medium heat for about 10 minutes, or until the cranberries begin to break down and release their juice.

When the water boils, add the fettuccine and cook according to the package instructions. Once cooked, drain the pasta, reserving some of the cooking water.

Add the pasta to the pan with the cranberries, mixing well to coat with the sauce. If necessary, add some cooking water to create a creamier consistency.

Finally, grate the black truffle over the pasta, add a pinch of nutmeg, and adjust salt and pepper. Garnish with fresh basil leaves and serve immediately.

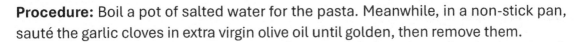

Benefits: Black truffle and cranberries give this recipe a unique and unexpected taste, in addition to having anti-inflammatory properties. A first course rich in fibers, vitamins, and minerals, ideal for a gourmet and healthy meal.

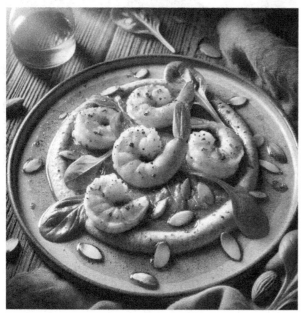

"Shrimp on Watercress Cream: A Riot of Flavors!"

Ingredients for 4 people:

400 grams of cleaned shrimp

150 grams of fresh watercress

200 ml of almond milk

1 clove of garlic

Extra virgin olive oil as needed

Salt and pepper to taste

Toasted almond flakes for garnish

Procedure: Start with the watercress cream. In a saucepan, bring the almond milk to a boil with a pinch of salt. Add the watercress and cook for 3-4 minutes. Transfer the contents to a blender and blend until you get a smooth and velvety cream.

Meanwhile, in a non-stick pan, sauté the garlic with a drizzle of olive oil. Add the shrimp and cook for about 2-3 minutes per side, until they turn pink and opaque.

To serve, spread a bed of watercress cream on the plates, lay the shrimp on top, and garnish with toasted almond flakes and a drizzle of extra virgin olive oil.

Benefits: This dish is a perfect balance of flavors and nutrients. The shrimp are a great source of lean protein and omega-3, useful for fighting inflammation. Watercress, with its antioxidant and anti-inflammatory properties, adds a touch of freshness and a unique flavor to the dish. Finally, almond milk and toasted almonds add a sweet and crunchy note, in addition to being an excellent source of vitamin E and monounsaturated fats, beneficial for heart health.

"Squid Ink Risotto with Pink Grapefruit Slices"

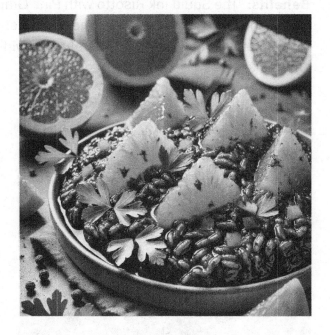

Ingredients for 4 people:

350g of Carnaroli rice

60g of squid ink

1l of fish stock

1 small pink grapefruit

1 small white onion

Extra virgin olive oil

Salt and pepper to taste

Fresh parsley for garnish

Procedure: Start by finely chopping the onion and sauté it in a little oil in a large pan. When the onion is transparent, add the rice and toast it for a couple of minutes.

Dilute the squid ink in a ladle of hot broth and add it to the rice, stirring well to color every grain. At this point, start adding the rest of the hot fish broth, a ladle at a time, stirring continuously.

While the rice cooks, peel the grapefruit and cut the flesh into thin slices, trying to remove the seeds.

When the risotto is cooked al dente, adjust the salt and pepper; then, plate up, decorating with slices of grapefruit and a sprinkling of freshly chopped parsley.

Benefits: "The Squid Ink Risotto with Pink Grapefruit Slices" offers a surprising mix of marine and citrus flavors. The ingredients used are known for their anti-inflammatory properties, with grapefruit providing vitamin C and the squid ink rich in Omega-3.

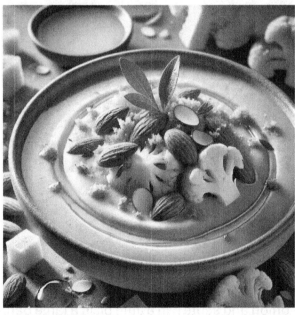

"Cauliflower and Curry Soup with Toasted Almond Crumble"

Ingredients for 4 people:

400g of cauliflower

1l of vegetable broth

2 teaspoons of curry powder

100g of almonds

Extra virgin olive oil

Salt and pepper to taste

Procedure: Start by toasting the almonds in a non-stick pan without oil. When they become golden, roughly chop them, and set aside.

Take the cauliflower, separate the florets, wash them, and put them in a pot with the vegetable broth. Cook until the cauliflower is very soft. Add the curry, salt, and pepper, and blend everything with an immersion blender until you get a smooth and creamy soup.

Serve the soup in individual bowls, sprinkle with the chopped toasted almonds, and drizzle with raw olive oil.

Benefits: "The Cauliflower and Curry Soup with Toasted Almond Crumble" is a sophisticated and nutritious first course. Cauliflower is an excellent natural anti-inflammatory, while curry is known for its antioxidant properties. Almonds, rich in vitamin E, complete this symphony of flavors and health benefits.

"Whole Grain Rice Lasagna with Ratatouille"

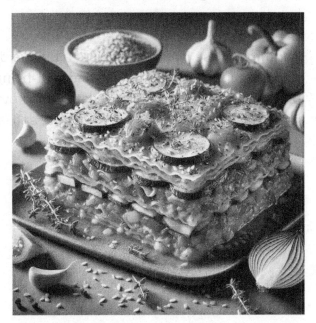

Ingredients for 4 people:

16 sheets of whole grain rice lasagna

2 small eggplants

2 zucchinis

2 red bell peppers

2 onions

4 cloves of garlic

800g of peeled tomatoes

4 tablespoons of extra virgin olive oil

Salt and pepper to taste

4 sprigs of fresh thyme

4 sprigs of fresh rosemary

Procedure: Start by cutting all the vegetables into small cubes. In a large pan, sauté the onion and garlic in oil, then add the other vegetables, peeled tomatoes, thyme, rosemary, salt, and pepper. Cook on low heat for about 30 minutes, until the vegetables are well cooked.

Meanwhile, cook the whole grain rice lasagna sheets according to the package instructions.

Once ready, take a baking dish and start layering the lasagna: one layer of lasagna, one layer of vegetables, and continue in this way until all ingredients are used up.

Bake at 180°C (356°F) for 15-20 minutes.

Benefits: These rice lasagnas are a unique dish that combines Italian and French traditions in a fusion of flavors and well-being. Whole grain rice is rich in fiber and promotes digestion, while vegetables provide a wide variety of vitamins and minerals. A dish that pleases the palate and is good for health!

"A Masterpiece of Nutrition and Flavor: Gourmet Main Courses"

Transform every recipe into a painting made of colors, lights, and shadows that, just like a landscape, can tell a story. Just as a photographer captures the most breathtaking landscapes, every gourmet dish captures attention and enchants, leaving an indelible mark in the memory of those who taste it.

Each recipe is a work of art, a masterpiece that expresses balance, symmetry, and harmony. As in a perfect photograph, every element finds its place, nothing is left to chance. The flavors blend into a culinary experience that delights the palate, nourishes the body, and caresses the soul.

From this perspective, creating a gourmet main course is like waiting for the perfect moment to take a picture, when the light is right, the subject is posed, and everything comes together to create something extraordinary. In this culinary framework, nutrition becomes flavor, and flavor becomes art.

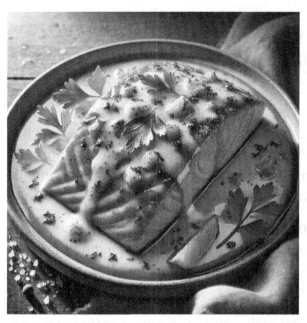

"Salmon Fillet in a Ginger Jacket"

Ingredients for 4 people:

4 salmon fillets (about 100g each)

60g of fresh ginger

200ml of coconut milk

The juice of 1 lemon

A bunch of fresh parsley

Salt and pepper to taste

Procedure: Preheat the oven to 180 degrees. Clean and grate the ginger, then chop it into small pieces.

In a blender, put the pieces of ginger, coconut milk, and lemon juice. Blend until you get a smooth sauce. Add salt and pepper to your taste.

Place the salmon fillets in a baking dish and pour the ginger sauce over them. Bake for 15-20 minutes, or until the salmon is well cooked but still juicy.

While the salmon is in the oven, wash and chop the fresh parsley. Once cooked, serve the salmon hot, garnished with the chopped parsley.

Voilà! Your "Salmon Fillet in a Ginger Jacket" is ready to be enjoyed!

Benefits: The benefits of this recipe are numerous. Salmon is rich in Omega-3s, which fight inflammation and promote heart health. Ginger, with its antioxidant and anti-inflammatory properties, further reinforces these virtues. A meal that not only delights the palate but also takes care of the body!

"Chicken Roll-up with Plums: An Anti-inflammatory Delight"

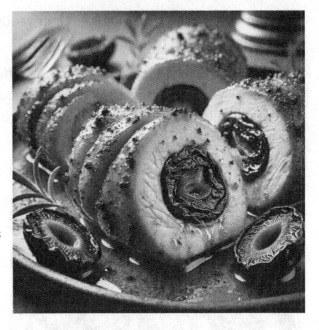

Ingredients for 4 people:

4 chicken breasts, about 100 grams each

16 pitted dried plums

1 teaspoon of turmeric powder

2 teaspoons of chopped fresh rosemary

Salt and pepper to taste

Extra virgin olive oil as needed

50 ml of balsamic vinegar

Kitchen twine for tying the roll-ups

Procedure: Start with the chicken. Open the chicken breasts like a book, without cutting them all the way through. Season the inside with a bit of salt, pepper, and turmeric.

Evenly distribute 4 dried plums on each opened chicken breast.

Gently roll up each chicken breast, making sure the plums stay inside. Tie the roll-ups with kitchen twine to keep them closed during cooking.

In a non-stick pan, heat a drizzle of olive oil. Add the chicken roll-ups and brown them on all sides. When the roll-ups are well browned, add the balsamic vinegar and rosemary, and if needed, a few tablespoons of water. Cover the pan and cook over medium heat for about 20 minutes. Once ready, let the roll-ups rest for a few minutes before removing the twine and slicing them.

Benefits: The chicken roll-ups with plums offer a balanced nutritional mix; the lean meat of the chicken together with the fiber-rich plums and anti-inflammatory turmeric combine to create a dish that is a true boon for health.

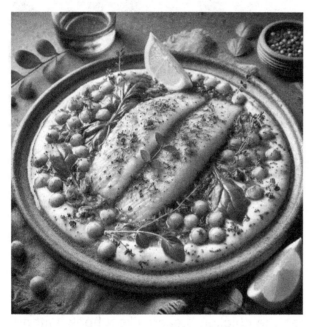

"Sole Fillets with Aromatic Herbs and Chickpea Cream: An Anti-inflammatory Gourmet Dream"

Ingredients for 4 people:

4 sole fillets, 150 grams each

1 organic lemon

A mix of fresh herbs (thyme, parsley, basil) to taste

400 grams of cooked chickpeas

2 cloves of garlic

Extra virgin olive oil as needed

Salt and pepper to taste

Procedure: Start with the chickpea cream. In a blender, combine the chickpeas, a pinch of salt, pepper, and a drizzle of extra virgin olive oil. Blend until you obtain a smooth and homogeneous cream.

Meanwhile, heat a drizzle of oil in a non-stick pan. Add the garlic and sauté until golden brown. Remove the garlic and add the sole fillets, cooking them for about 3-4 minutes per side. Just before finishing cooking, add the chopped herbs and the grated zest of the lemon.

To serve, spread a bed of chickpea cream on the plates, lay the sole fillets on top, and garnish with a drizzle of extra virgin olive oil.

Benefits: This dish offers a perfect combination of lean proteins from the fish, fibers and plant proteins from the chickpeas, and a dose of antioxidants from the aromatic herbs. Sole is a lean fish with low fat and calorie content but rich in high-quality proteins. The fresh herbs, besides adding flavor, are an excellent source of vitamins and antioxidants. Finally, chickpeas, rich in fibers, proteins, and anti-inflammatory substances, complete this delicious and healthy gourmet dish.

"Baked Octopus with Jerusalem Artichoke Sauce: A Gourmet Harmony of Sea and Land"

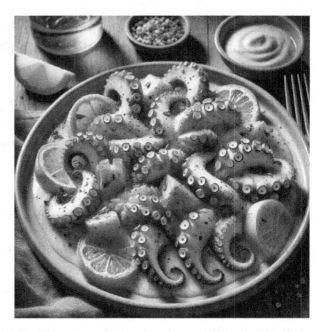

Ingredients for 4 people:

400 grams of cleaned octopus

500 grams of Jerusalem artichokes

2 cloves of garlic

2 sprigs of fresh thyme

Extra virgin olive oil as needed

Salt and pepper to taste

Juice of 1 lemon

Vegetable broth as needed

Procedure: Begin with preparing the octopus. Bring a pot of water to a boil, immerse the octopus, and cook for about 40 minutes. Once cooked, let it cool in the cooking water.

Meanwhile, peel the Jerusalem artichokes and cut them into pieces. In a pan, heat a drizzle of olive oil, add the garlic, and let it golden. Add the Jerusalem artichokes, season with salt and pepper, and add the thyme. After a few minutes, cover the Jerusalem artichokes with vegetable broth and let them cook until soft.

Once cooked, blend the Jerusalem artichokes with an immersion mixer, adding broth until you achieve a creamy sauce. Adjust with salt and pepper.

Cut the octopus into pieces and place them on a baking tray. Season with a drizzle of oil, salt, pepper, and the lemon juice. Bake in a preheated oven at 200 degrees for about 10-15 minutes until the octopus becomes crispy.

Spread the Jerusalem artichoke sauce on the bottom of the plates, lay the octopus on top, and serve.

Benefits: This dish offers a delicate balance between the sea flavor of the octopus and the uniqueness of Jerusalem artichokes, a root rich in fibers and with anti-inflammatory properties. The addition of lemon provides a refreshing note that perfectly ties the ingredients together.

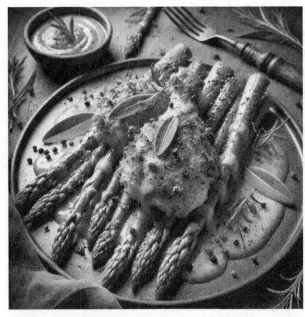

"Herb-Crusted Chicken with Wild Asparagus and Turmeric Sauce"

Ingredients for 4 people:

400 grams of deboned chicken

300 grams of wild asparagus

2 tablespoons of turmeric

2 cloves of garlic

Aromatic herbs (rosemary, sage, thyme) to taste

Extra virgin olive oil as needed

Salt and pepper to taste

200 ml of vegetable broth

Juice of 1 lemon

200 grams of Greek yogurt

Procedure: Prepare the marinade for the chicken with a mix of chopped aromatic herbs, salt, pepper, and oil. Immerse the chicken and let it rest in the refrigerator for at least 2 hours. Meanwhile, clean the asparagus by removing the hardest part of the stem. Sauté them in a pan with a drizzle of oil, a clove of garlic, salt, and pepper. Prepare the sauce by mixing the yogurt with turmeric, lemon juice, salt, and pepper. Cook the chicken in the oven at 180°C (356°F) for about 20 minutes, or until it is golden and crispy. Serve the chicken on a bed of wild asparagus and finish with a drizzle of turmeric sauce.

Benefits: Turmeric, with its well-known anti-inflammatory properties, is the star of this special sauce that pairs perfectly with the tenderness of the chicken and the freshness of the asparagus. A dish rich in flavors and vitamins such as vitamin A from the asparagus and various B vitamins from the chicken, not to mention the powerful antioxidants contained in turmeric. A true triumph of health and flavor.

"The Art of Indulgence: Gourmet Desserts"

Gourmet anti-inflammatory desserts strike the perfect balance between health and pleasure. They represent a culinary art form that embraces both functionality and creativity, turning each bite into a full sensory experience. These delights demonstrate that taste does not have to be sacrificed for a healthy and mindful diet. Elegance, innovation, and well-being are woven into every creation, transforming dessert into a key player in a conscious and rewarding dietary approach.

"Gourmet Licorice Semifreddo: An Anti-inflammatory Delight"

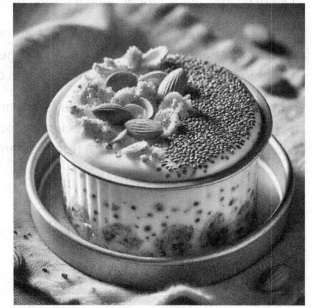

Ingredients for 4 people:

300g natural Greek yogurt

50g fresh licorice root, grated

4 tablespoons of raw honey

100g whole grain biscuits, crumbled

50g toasted almonds

2 teaspoons chia seeds

Procedure: Start by finely grating the fresh licorice root. This will add a distinctive and therapeutic flavor to our semifreddo.

Mix the Greek yogurt with the honey in a bowl. The honey not only adds sweetness but brings powerful antioxidant properties. Add the grated licorice and mix well. Put this mixture in the fridge to rest for at least an hour, allowing the licorice to infuse the yogurt.

Crumble the whole grain biscuits and toast the almonds. The almonds add crunchiness and a wonderful contrast in texture, while the biscuits provide the base for our semifreddo.

Once your yogurt mix has rested, gently incorporate the chia seeds. These seeds are a potent source of antioxidants and give an interesting texture to the dessert.

To assemble the semifreddo, use molds. Layer crumbled biscuits, the yogurt mix, and toasted almonds alternately. Repeat until the molds are filled, finishing with a layer of yogurt. Freeze for at least 4 hours, or until the semifreddo is solidified.

Before serving, let the semifreddos rest at room temperature for 10 minutes. This dessert is a true triumph of flavors and wellness, combining the natural sweetness of honey with the intensity of licorice and the crunchiness of almonds.

Benefits: This licorice semifreddo is full of anti-inflammatory properties thanks to the licorice and honey, as well as being a good source of fiber and antioxidants due to the chia seeds and almonds. A true masterpiece of taste and health.

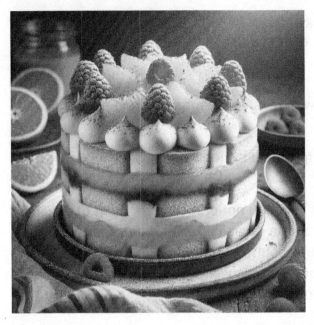

"Orange Vanilla Delight: The Anti-inflammatory Ricotta Tiramisu"

Ingredients for 4 servings:

500g of low-fat ricotta

4 tablespoons of raw honey

400g of whole wheat ladyfingers (savoiardi)

4 fresh peaches

200g of fresh raspberries

Juice of 2 large oranges

1 teaspoon of vanilla extract

Dark chocolate shavings for decoration

Procedure: Start with the ricotta cream: Blend the ricotta with honey until you achieve a smooth and creamy consistency. This ricotta base provides a light flavor and creamy texture, as well as beneficial anti-inflammatory properties.

Prepare the fruits: Wash the peaches and raspberries. Dice the peaches and set aside some whole raspberries for decoration. Blend the remaining raspberries with the diced peaches to create a fresh fruit puree.

Create the soaking liquid: Mix the orange juice with vanilla extract. This aromatic blend adds a refreshing and flavorful twist to the tiramisu.

Assemble the tiramisu: Dip the ladyfingers quickly in the orange-vanilla mixture and lay them in a layer at the bottom of a baking dish. Spread a layer of ricotta cream over the ladyfingers, followed by a generous amount of fruit puree. Repeat the layering until all ingredients are used, ending with a final layer of ricotta cream.

Final touches: Garnish the top layer with reserved raspberries and dark chocolate shavings for a rich, decorative finish.

Chill and set: Refrigerate the tiramisu for at least 2 hours to allow the flavors to meld together beautifully.

Benefits: This Orange Vanilla Ricotta Tiramisu not only offers a burst of delightful flavors but also boasts health benefits. The combination of antioxidant-rich fruits, anti-inflammatory honey, and the heart-healthy fats from dark chocolate make this dessert not just indulgent but also good for your well-being. Enjoy a dessert that's both delicious and nurturing to your body.

"Green Joy: Pistachio, Almond, and Hazelnut Semifreddo"

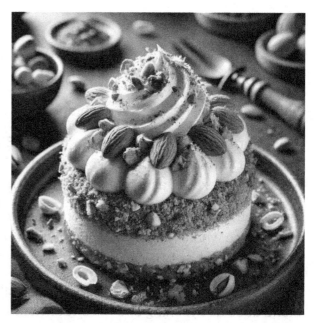

Ingredients for 4 servings, a 22cm cake tin:

200g of unsalted pistachios

200g of unsalted almonds

200g of roasted hazelnuts

500ml of plant-based cream

200g of agave syrup or honey

Grated zest of 1 organic lemon

2 teaspoons of vanilla extract

5 crumbled walnuts for decoration

Procedure: Begin by roasting the pistachios, almonds, and hazelnuts in the oven at 180°C for 10 minutes, or until they become golden and fragrant. Allow them to cool completely.

Prepare the biscuit base by blending 100g of each type of nut in a food processor until you have a sandy mixture. Add 100g of agave syrup or honey and mix until uniform. Press the mixture into the base of the cake tin and place it in the refrigerator to cool.

Blend the remaining 100g of each type of nut until you obtain a smooth and spreadable cream. Add the lemon zest and vanilla extract and mix until well combined.

Whip the plant-based cream until soft peaks form and gently fold it into the nut cream. Pour the mixture over the biscuit base and smooth the surface with a spatula. Place the semifreddo in the freezer for at least 4 hours, or until it has set.

Remove the semifreddo from the freezer 10-15 minutes before serving to allow it to soften slightly. Garnish with chopped walnuts and almonds, and decorate as you wish.

Benefits: The ingredients in this cake are sources of vitamins E and B, minerals such as magnesium, iron, zinc, and contain polyunsaturated fatty acids that help combat inflammation. A healthy and nutritious gourmet delight!

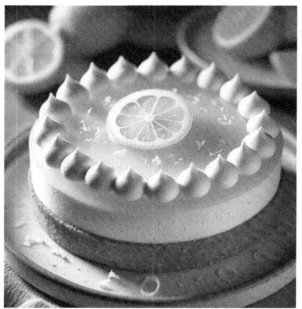

"Lemon and Ginger Tart with Almond and Date Base"

Ingredients for a 22cm tart:

200g almonds

150g Medjool dates, pitted

A pinch of salt

For the filling:

Juice and zest of 3 organic lemons

1 teaspoon of grated fresh ginger

200ml agave syrup

100ml almond milk

3 tablespoons cornstarch

Procedure: Begin by preparing the base. Grind the almonds in a food processor until sandy in texture. Add the dates and salt, blending until a dough forms. Press the dough onto the base of a tart pan and refrigerate to cool.

For the filling, combine lemon juice and zest, grated ginger, agave syrup, and almond milk in a saucepan. Bring to a boil over medium heat. Add the cornstarch and stir constantly until thickened. Pour the filling over the almond and date base and chill in the refrigerator for at least 3 hours, or until set.

Benefits: This tart offers a rich mix of vitamin C, fiber, and antioxidants thanks to the citrus and ginger. Almonds provide a good dose of vitamin E and protein, while dates add natural sweetness and fiber.

"Black Volcanoes: Dark Chocolate Soufflé with a Heart of Sour Cherries"

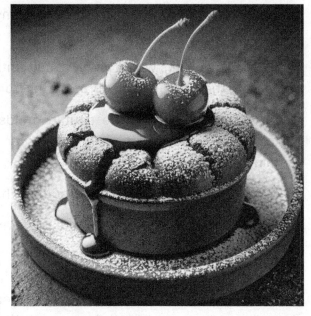

Ingredients for 4 servings:

120g dark chocolate (at least 70% cocoa)

100g sour cherries in syrup (no added sugar)

3 tablespoons of sour cherry juice

80g lactose-free butter

60g spelt flour

80g coconut sugar

3 large eggs, separated

1 teaspoon of vanilla extract

A pinch of salt

Icing sugar for decoration

Procedure: Preheat the oven to 200°C (392°F). Grease and flour four soufflé molds.

Melt the chocolate and butter in a bain-marie, stirring until smooth. Remove from the heat and add the flour, coconut sugar, sour cherry juice, and vanilla extract. Mix well.

In another bowl, whip the egg yolks until foamy. Gradually incorporate the chocolate mixture, continuing to stir.

Whisk the egg whites with a pinch of salt until soft peaks form. Gently fold the egg whites into the chocolate mixture, stirring from the bottom up to keep the air in.

Divide the batter among the soufflé molds, filling them about halfway. Add a tablespoon of sour cherries in the center of each mold, then cover with the remaining batter.

Bake for 12-15 minutes, or until the soufflés have risen and are golden.

Serve immediately, dusted with icing sugar and a couple of sour cherries on top of each soufflé.

Benefits: These black volcanoes take you on a journey of sweetness: the dark chocolate provides antioxidants, the sour cherries anti-inflammatory benefits, while the coconut sugar and spelt flour enrich the dessert with fiber, for a surprisingly gourmet finale.

Quote: *"A well-made cocktail can really take you away." - Dean Martin.*

CHAPTER 15

"Anti-Inflammatory Cocktails and Appetizers"

In this vibrant universe of cocktails and appetizers, a cosmopolitan theater of colors, flavors, and emotions unfolds. Here, every cocktail is a symphony of sensations, an experience that invites discovery and sharing. From the warm and welcoming tones of the drinks to the intense and vibrant colors of the appetizers, every element is designed to create a harmony of taste and well-being.

This is not just about food and drinks, but about an art, a universal language that brings people together. A well-prepared cocktail is a work of art, an explosion of flavors that dance on the palate, perfectly accompanied by an assortment of appetizers, each with its own distinct personality and taste.

On one hand, the cocktail is emotion, euphoria, the starting point of an unforgettable evening. On the other, the appetizers are comfort, the pleasure of discovering and savoring new flavors. Both represent the celebration of moments of conviviality, an invitation to slow down, to take the time to taste and appreciate the small pleasures of life. All of this, of course, with an eye always on well-being, because the true art lies in finding the right balance between taste and health.

"Tropical Party: Sun Cocktail & Sea Delights"

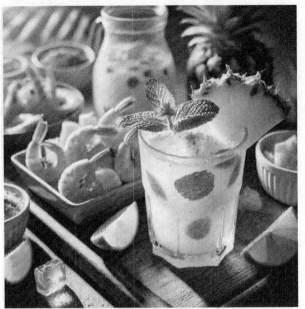

Ingredients for 4 people:

Juice of 8 fresh limes

480 ml of pineapple juice

8 tablespoons of turmeric powder

A large handful of fresh mint leaves

For the Sea Delights, you will need:

500g of shrimp

2 cloves of garlic

Juice of 1 lemon

2 tablespoons of olive oil

1 teaspoon of grated fresh ginger

Procedure for the Cocktail: Mix the lime juice, pineapple, and turmeric in a blender until smooth. Pour the cocktail into chilled glasses and garnish with a mint leaf.

Procedure for the Sea Delights: Heat the olive oil in a pan, add the garlic and ginger, and sauté for a minute. Add the shrimp and cook until they turn pink. Squeeze the lemon juice over and serve.

Benefits: The cocktail and snacks offer an abundance of antioxidants and anti-inflammatory nutrients. The combination of pineapple, turmeric, and ginger brings benefits known for their anti-inflammatory properties. A delight for the palate with health in mind.

"Vibrant Party: Happiness Cocktail & Earthy Crisps"

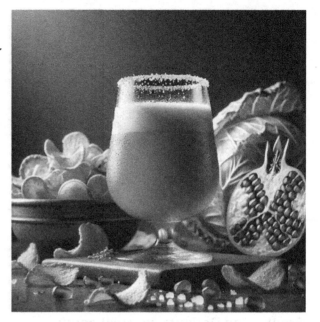

Ingredients for 4 people:

800 ml of pomegranate juice

800 ml of peach juice

4 teaspoons of honey

For the Earthy Crisps, you will need:

200 g of carrots

200 g of cabbage

Extra virgin olive oil

Sea salt

Procedure for the Cocktail: In a pitcher, mix the pomegranate juice and peach juice. Add the honey and stir until completely dissolved. Keep refrigerated until ready to serve.

Procedure for the Earthy Crisps: Wash and cut the carrots and cabbage into thin strips. Heat the olive oil in a pan and fry the vegetables over medium-high heat until they become crispy. Sprinkle with sea salt.

Benefits: This combination of cocktail and crisps offers a range of vitamins and minerals, contributing to an anti-inflammatory approach to nutrition. A feast for both the palate and health!

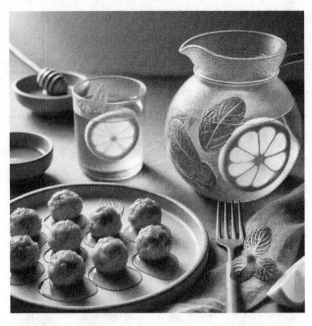

"Zen Harmony: Green Tea Infusion & Citrus Chicken Meatballs"

Ingredients for 4 people:

4 tablespoons of loose green tea leaves

1 liter of water

2 tablespoons of acacia honey

A bunch of fresh mint (about 15-20 leaves)

Juice of 2 lemons

For the Citrus Chicken Meatballs, you will need:

500g of ground chicken

Zest of 2 organic lemons

Soy sauce, as needed

Procedure for the Cocktail: Bring the liter of water to a boil. Once boiling, turn off the heat and add the loose green tea leaves and mint. Let it steep for 5-10 minutes.

Strain the tea into a pitcher, removing the leaves and mint, add the lemon juice and mix well. Add the acacia honey and stir until completely dissolved.

Cool the cocktail in the refrigerator for at least an hour before serving. Serve the cocktail chilled, adding ice cubes if desired. For an extra touch of color and freshness, garnish the glasses with a mint leaf.

Procedure for the Citrus Chicken Meatballs: In a bowl, mix the ground chicken with the lemon zest. Form small meatballs and cook in a non-stick pan with a little olive oil. Serve with a drizzle of soy sauce.

Benefits: This combination offers antioxidants from green tea and lean proteins from chicken, coupled with the refreshing aroma of lemon. An explosion of flavors and well-being.

"Orange Sunset Cocktail & Crunchy Party"

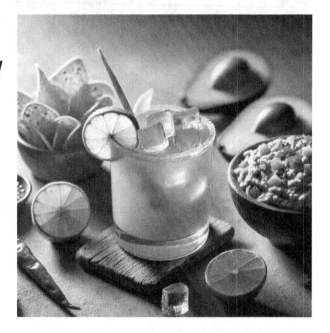

Ingredients for 4 people:

12 fresh carrots

4 oranges

4 cm of fresh ginger

Ice

For the Tortillas with Guacamole:

8 corn tortillas

4 ripe avocados

2 limes

Salt and pepper to taste

1 red chili pepper

2 ripe tomatoes

Procedure for the Cocktail: Juice the carrots, oranges, and ginger in a juicer. Chill the obtained juice in the refrigerator. Serve the cocktail with ice cubes.

Procedure for the Tortillas with Guacamole: Cut the avocados in half and remove the pit. Mash the pulp with a fork and add the juice of the limes, salt, pepper, and the chopped chili pepper. Dice the tomatoes and add them to the guacamole. Serve the guacamole with the corn tortillas.

Benefits: This meal offers vitamins A, B, C, E, and K, fiber, potassium, and antioxidants, which support heart health and vision, and reduce inflammation. A mix of well-being and flavor.

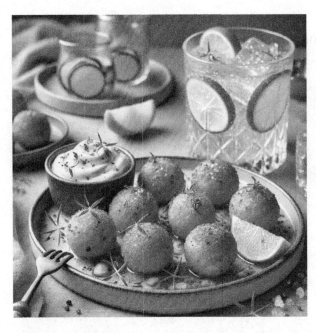

"Golden Ocean Temptations"

Ingredients for 4 people:

2 large cucumbers

1L of sparkling water

Ice

For the Salmon Balls:

600g of fresh salmon

1 bunch of aromatic herbs (dill, parsley, basil)

1 teaspoon of powdered saffron

Salt and pepper to taste

Ingredients for the Exotic Cream:

200g of Greek yogurt

Juice and zest of 1 lime

Salt to taste

Procedure for the Cocktail: Slice the cucumbers thinly and place them in a pitcher. Add the sparkling water and stir. Chill the cocktail in the refrigerator. Serve with ice cubes.

Procedure for the Salmon Balls: Finely chop the salmon and herbs. Add the saffron, salt, and pepper. Form small balls and bake in the oven at 180°C (356°F) for 15 minutes.

For the exotic cream, mix the Greek yogurt with the lime juice and zest and a pinch of salt.

Benefits: The cocktail is rich in vitamins and antioxidants, while the salmon balls provide high-quality proteins, omega-3, and vitamins. A perfect mix for health and taste.

Thank you immensely for joining me on this fascinating journey through pages full of flavors, stories, and new discoveries. Your interest, commitment, and passion have made this journey even more captivating. Every small step you take, every change you embrace, builds a brick on the road to your well-being. Do not fear obstacles; we face them to grow, to become stronger. I know you are capable of great things, as you've already shown by following me this far.

Food is art, medicine, love. Learning to respect it, love it, and use its qualities for your well-being can lead to a healthy and tasty life. However, always remember to consult a nutrition professional or a dietitian for personalized and expert advice.

I wish you a bright future filled with happiness, success, and health. Always be proud of your progress and continue pursuing your dreams with fervor and determination.

"And as the unforgettable Audrey Hepburn once said, 'The most important thing is to enjoy your food.' Savor your Life!

If you think you enjoyed this book and it helped you feel better, I would be extremely grateful if you could share your experience by leaving a review on Amazon.

Your words will not only help me improve, but they could also help other people in their choice.

Your opinion matters!

Thank you very much!

Jenni Serges

Notes:

Made in the USA
Monee, IL
06 November 2024

69511464R10175